# The Prince and the PMS

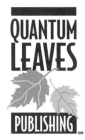

QUANTUM
LEAVES

PUBLISHING SM

ISBN-10: 0-9761526-1-4
ISBN-13: 978-0-9761526-1-3

First Edition. Printed in the United States of America.

BOOK DESIGN by TRACY STEVENS
CARTOONS by TURONNY FUAD/www.poggiwoggi.com
COVER ILLUSTRATIONS©CHUCK GONZALES/www.artscounselinc.com
COVER DESIGN by JOHN COSTA, New Orleans

Published by Quantum Leaves Publishing℠
Del Mar, California.
www.theprincessandthepms.com
www.quantumleaves.com

# With thanks to:

Jessica for the support and encouragement,
Audrey and David McKnight for their artistic skills and Ellen
Stiefler for keeping us on the right legal path

Tilak for helping us to be mindful

Bob, Joshua, Drew and Logan, the home team, for all the
laughter, light and love along the way

Dad, Ava, Splinky and Charger for
their boundless love and support

# Introduction

You don't know it yet, but I'm your new best buddy. I'm about to make the impossible possible, the out-of-control under control, and out-of-control sex possible! Have I got your attention?

After a lengthy bachelorhood, which included an engagement, rebound dead-ends, and live-in disasters that stopped short of restraining orders and concealed weapon permits, I've compiled everything I learned in this book. More specifically, I found a way to outsmart my lifelong archenemy and the "end zone" for my past relationships: PMS.

*The Prince and the PMS* is the result of my lifesaving research. I figure it's my guy duty to pass along what I learned to other suffering brothers since I credit the techniques in this book for my finally settling down – without settling.

That's right. The advice in *The Prince and the PMS* led me to my soulmate. Without strategies, such as the PMS Red Flag warning system and others within these pages, there's no chance in hell I'd walk down the plank, I mean, aisle. Mike Myers summarized how I used to feel in *Wayne's World*: "Marriage is punishment for shoplifting in some countries." But now, I'm ready to take the plunge.

PMS is real, and it literally cramps the style of millions of women and anyone within 10 city blocks. Living with PMS – even by association – can turn your life into a monthly low-budget, horror

flick: Nightmare on YOUR Street!  It's a whopping and creepy 12 times a year when you feel like you've entered the wrong house; where the female face you (normally) love is grossly disfigured by rage, tears and looniness; where one stupid word causes an atomic explosion, chocolate is the Holy Grail and a bottle of tequila seems like a reasonable remedy – for you!

Secondhand PMS, a term destined for infamy, can put a stranglehold on your relationships with mothers, sisters, wives, girlfriends, coworkers and flight attendants. It's a plague that has left countless comrades with estrogen-dripping shrapnel in their hind quarters, asking: "Where is the air raid drill, exit strategy and/or manual for this epidemic?" The answer: Right here!

In your hands you hold the "magic remote" that changes the channel on chaos and tunes in a happier, more peaceful life.  You'll learn to tinker with the way you confront the Premenstrual Terminator wearing your old sweatshirt. Like a clogged garbage disposal, you can fix this!

So, grab a cold one and turn the page to your future...a future without PMS winning home advantage!

(For those of you who haven't read anything since installing your big screens, there are plenty of cartoons, too.)

— Brian Young

# Contents

# A Note to Our Princes

PMS or IRS? It's a toss up which set of initials strikes more terror in the hearts of red-blooded males. We'll bet that given a choice, nearly all sane men would gladly take on a tax audit rather than confront a woman with raging premenstrual syndrome.

Behind every woman with PMS is a guy like you: a bad-ass bubba with a 300-horsepower engine or a flaming outdoor grill, who regresses to a girly-man when staring into the bloodshot eyes of Cruella de Drill Sergeant. Like the road to hell, efforts at PMS management may be paved with good intentions; yet, even the toughest among us feels defenseless against the premenstrual pummeling we endure.

Next time you exclaim,"What the #%*@!?" pick up this book and remind yourself that you have brothers, comrades in arms battling the same enemy: PMS. In other words, you're not alone. More importantly, there are ways to make things better when you're face to face with the Twinkie®-fueled she-devil. Take our quiz, "Know Thy Enemy: PMS" following this introduction to find out what type of PMS you're living with and what you can do to combat monthly hormonal harassment.

You might have assumed that having a penis excludes you from PMS. Sorry! Secondhand smoke may kill you, but "secondhand PMS" makes you suffer every month for 30 years or so! *The Prince and the PMS* provides male victims with the help they need to balance on an estrogen-slick tightrope – or at least gives them a running start to get the hell out!

*The Prince and the PMS* offers guy guidance, or *guy*dance, such as: Only tell "on the rag" jokes in a secure environment. Translation: NO WOMEN AROUND. Why? the suicidal among you ask. While a woman is "PMSing" – a verb that will eventually earn a spot in the dictionary – she has no sense of humor. Memorize that. Say it like a mantra. Tattoo it backwards on your forehead.

*So, why do they call it PMS? Answer: Because whiny-ass, cuckoo for Cocoa Puffs®, bloated bi-atch is a tongue-twister.*

Granted, the jokes are hard to resist. But, if you're committed to make any relationship with the opposite sex work – or just need to be committed – then ixnay on the okesjay until menopause (or as we like to call it, "global warming part 2"). Doesn't matter if the swollen, achy women you know find some humor in it; zip it, watch your back and bone up on what you're up against in "Just the Facts, Man" on page 27.

We cut through all the research and the pop psychology for a reality check: PMS is a fact of life, deal with it...or move to Alaska where men outnumber women 2 to 1. What women feel during the days leading up to their periods is about as pleasant as an extra large, cold catheter. From pain to depression, loss of self-esteem to insomnia, women exist in a state ranging from mild annoyance to the Bride of Chucky during PMS. So, do yourself a favor and learn how to work around "womanliness" by planning

ahead – proposals, barbeques, vasectomies – anything you were hoping to look back on fondly (see "PMS Alert" on page 43).

On the flip side of this book, those who have uteruses will find page after page of relationship-saving suggestions on how to minimize PMS and its disturbing effects. You might even want to do a little "bathroom" reading and check out her half of the book to support her battle. After all, you'll benefit as much from her efforts as she will.

So, instead of gearing up for a monthly confrontation with PMS, the mother of all opponents, figure out how to lessen your exposure while appearing to be a sensitive, caring guy. In between the laughs and enlightenment, we'll show you how. You'll be thanking the woman who threw this book at you in no time.

# Know Thy Enemy: PMS

More emotion-packed than a World Series 10th inning, more terrifying than the phrase "I'm late" from a girl who looks vaguely familiar, and more death-defying than outrunning pissed-off Spanish bulls, PMS whips the biggest, baddest and brightest among us. Like a rash, it appears suddenly, gets worse before it gets better and, depending upon the gross-out factor, makes being seen in public a problem.

When PMS drops the "B" (rhymes with "pitch") bomb, monogamy seems downright cruel and Ms. Right becomes Ms. Who the Hell Is That? before your very eyes. Want to find out more about this stranger who visits monthly? Take the following quiz to discover what type of PMS you're both suffering from.

## During certain days of the month...

1.  ...it feels as if you've entered the twilight zone because:
    a. nothing you say is right
    b. she cries for no apparent reason
    c. you haven't a clue what the argument is about
    d. she goes from delirium to despair in an instant
    e. your belongings are on the front lawn

2.  ...her most prominent symptoms are:
    a. groaning and moaning
    b. breasts the size of Volkswagens®
    c. male-bashing marathons with her girlfriends
    d. zero tolerance levels for...EVERYTHING!
    e. all of the above

3. ...she's most likely to say/scream:

    a. "You're not here for me emotionally."
    b. "Who ate my (enter ANY food item here)?"
    c. "Why me?"
    d. "Hold me. Don't touch me. I love you. Get out!"
    e. "My mother was right about you!"

4. ...she spends most of her time:

    a. brushing off crumbs from her sweats
    b. convinced she's pregnant
    c. shouting ultimatums
    d. predicting the apocalypse
    e. packing

5. ...you earn the most brownie points for:

    a. giving her a brownie
    b. mopping the floor
    c. complimenting her
    d. clipping her toenails
    e. increasing your life insurance

6. ...the emotional climate at home can be described as:

    a. a cold front
    b. a flash flood
    c. a high pressure system
    d. a dense fog
    e. emotional climate?

7. ...you can reduce her symptoms by:

    a. giving her a massage
    b. kissing her ass
    c. hiding all mirrors and reflective surfaces
    d. leaving
    e. mashing an Ambien® into her second dinner

## 8. ...her sex drive:

a. peaks at inopportune times (e.g., the 7th game of the NBA® finals)
b. starts with 45 minutes of pleading and ends with a banana split
c. depends on the TV lineup
d. fluctuates with her personalities
e. what sex drive?

## 9. ...arguments are most frequently about:

a. your driving
b. your insensitivity
c. your nose hair
d. your existence
e. the toilet seat

## 10. ...the magic words are:

a. "I'm sorry."
b. "Have you been working out?"
c. "I finally fixed the _____."
d. "How 'bout some new shoes?"
e. "You're right. I'm an idiot."

# Answers

Now add up how many "a" answers you gave, how many "b" answers, etc. and turn the page to see who you've been living with every month. It's possible – in fact, likely – for your partner to present more than one "personality," so be sure to read all relevant and terrifying descriptions.

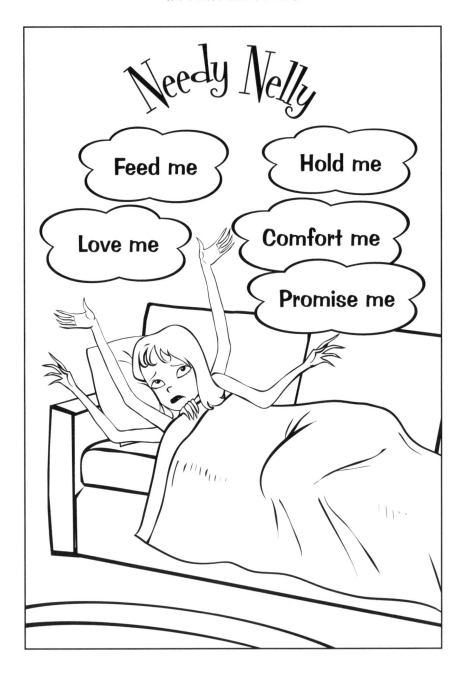

# Needy Nelly (mostly "a" answers)

Needy Nelly's favorite chant is "If you loved me you'd..." She issues more "tests" than an STD clinic. The hoops you have to jump through to keep the peace require the patience of a saint and faith that the crap will end when her period begins. But first, you must endure her analysis of your emotional shortcomings. Your premenstrual hell begins with the four words dreaded by men everywhere: "Let's talk about it."

A Needy Nelly expects you to understand what she wants and needs without her saying anything at all. She'll lie in wait then pounce when you don't read her mind. She can't fathom why massaging her feet isn't as much a treat for you as it is for her. Her PMS-induced fantasy involves you doing one or more of the following: putting the toilet seat down, taking out the trash without being asked, wearing a tool belt. In her fragile mind, these acts are proof positive that you care.

**The good news:** She's attentive.
**The bad news:** She always sends you for the tampons.

## What you can do:

With Needy Nelly, a good PMS offensive strike can reduce the torture. Lay the compliments and "yes, dears" on thick, and you'll be able to spend more time watching ESPN® and less time talking about any dreaded "R" words (Relationship, Responsibility or Romance – choose your poison).

Begin each PMS day by trying not to gag on, "Honey, what's the one thing I can do to make your life easier?" Think of it as a mouth condom designed to prevent undesirable verbal leakage

(a.k.a. speaking). You're also setting boundaries by offering to do one thing to help, instead of sinking into the black hole of neediness and agreeing to a list of things that would blow your whole day. Of course, you could choose to leave the house before she wakes up. That way, you don't have to say anything at all.

In the words of Austin Powers' Dr. Evil, "Throw her a frickin' bone." If she's trying to kick coffee, bring her some herbal tea. If she's trying to lose weight, choke down a few sprouts in front of her (you can grab a Big Mac® while you're out, but don't forget the breath mints!). Encourage her efforts by noticing – or pretending you notice – a difference in her appearance and behavior, but be careful not to imply that there was anything wrong with her before. Flattery such as "You look great today" is safe. On the other hand, "Jeez, you look a whole lot better than you did this time last month" will end in searing pain to your groin.

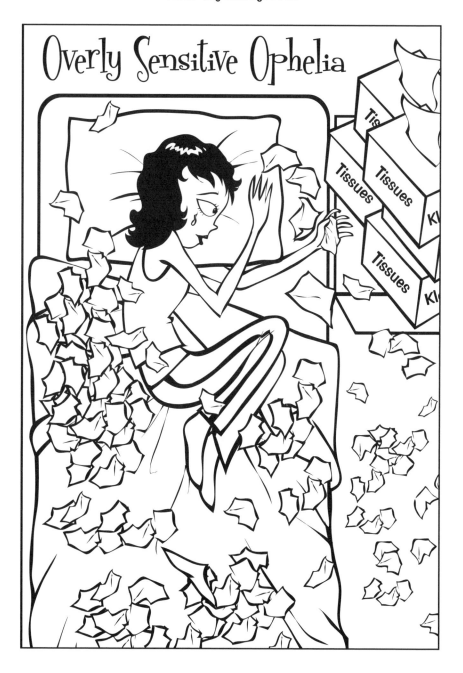

# Overly Sensitive Ophelia (mostly "b" answers)

Not only are her breasts tender, but so is her mental health. You're forced to walk on eggshells to avoid scrambling her delicate premenstrual psychological state. Each month, the first sign of PMS is her insistence that it isn't "that time" again. "I'm not emotional! I'm not overreacting!" Ophelia's inclined to shriek while flinging herself onto the bed or waving a steak knife for emphasis.

She accuses you of snoring on purpose because you're plotting to keep her awake. Or, she's certain you leave dirty clothes on the floor or forget to flush to punish her. "What do you want from me?" she wails when you ask her if the mail came or if she remembered to buy you shaving cream. "Am I supposed to do everything? All I do is give, give, give!" plays on a loop in her weepy head.

**The good news:** She's so emotionally drained she forgets to send you for the tampons.

**The bad news:** The only wet spot is from her tears.

# What you can do:

She feels unappreciated, so watch out! Your best bet is to stiff-arm PMS and steer clear of her crying fits and pity parties. When Ophelia ODs on hormones, it's all about her. You, on the other hand, are the loser staring up at a plummeting piano in her Looney Tunes® adventure.

Ophelia's arrival should signal your departure. This would be a great time to schedule after-hours meetings or late-night poker games. Never, and we mean **NEVER**, try to reason with her during PMS. Ask about her demon-double later in the month when its fangs disappear. Do it through clenched teeth if you have to, but convince her you're interested in what she goes through every month.

Above all, she needs validation. Tell her that the house is spotless, the meatloaf was phenomenal and she looks like a supermodel. Reinforce her self-worth with declarations like, "I am one lucky guy" or "That was the best sex I ever had" – assuming, of course, that Ophelia gave it up between breakdowns.

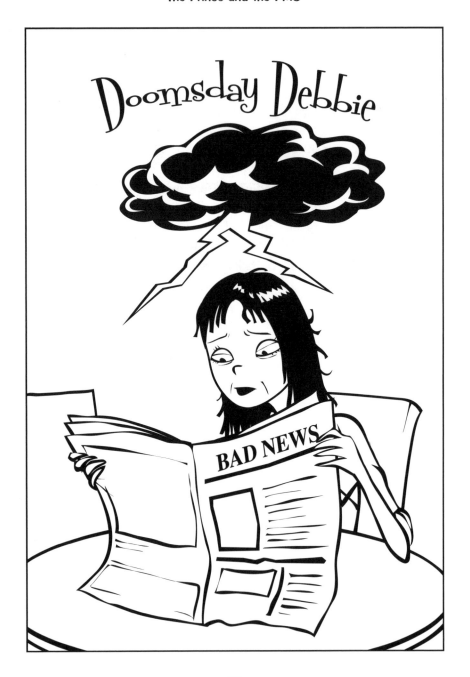

# Doomsday Debbie (mostly "c" answers)

When PMS strikes, this woman's long, drawn-out sighs can be heard from a block away. Though you try your damnedest to avoid asking about the cause of this annoying habit, ignoring it would be like walking past a murder scene without inquiring "what happened?" Of course, asking her what's wrong invites her to actually tell you!

Doomsday Debbie worries about worrying. She dreams up worst case scenarios then spouts statistics on the likelihood of them occurring. The only light at the end of the tunnel is the oncoming PMS train – and you're tied to the tracks. The grass is never greener because all vegetation will soon be burned by the hole in the ozone and global warming will render Earth a virtual fireball disintegrating all life forms. That is if an onslaught of killer bees doesn't get you first.

**The good news:** She's occupied.
**The bad news:** It's all about bad news.

# What you can do:

Short of installing a panic room, prepare for the approaching hormone hurricane by stockpiling ibuprofen for her and scotch for you – then plotting your escape route, just in case.

Help yourself while helping her by countering Debbie's "what if..." ramblings with doses of reality. Point out the positives in her life: family, career, wall-to-wall carpeting, YOU, etc. Reassure her that Armageddon is just a movie and all models are airbrushed.

Try to muster a little sympathy. Think of your worst performance anxiety nightmares. You know the ones: Carmen Electra and her hottest friends are ready and willing, but you're not able. It's kind of like that for her but without the breasts, short skirts and stilettos. Sucks, doesn't it?

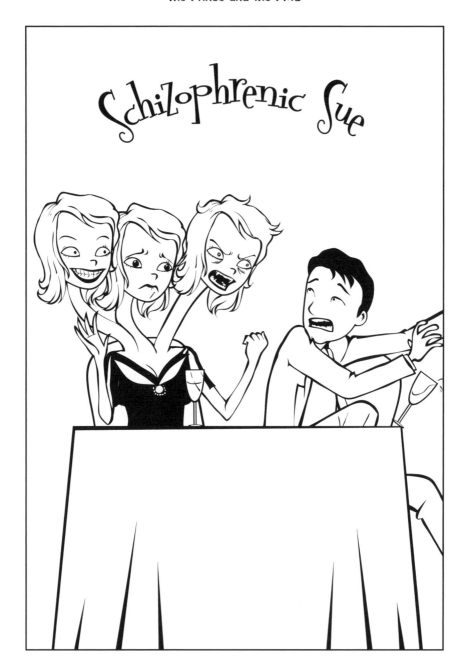

# Schizophrenic Sue (mostly "d" answers)

Is there a 5-foot female hormone with three heads messing with your sanity every 28 days or so? Does the lady in your life switch emotional channels faster than a TV remote under the thigh of a Weight Watcher's® client? Does she dare you to respond, bawl when you do, break things intentionally, then apologize profusely? If so, Schizophrenic Sue is most likely the culprit.

Her moods take twists and turns faster than a Porsche® on a mountain road. This divided diva is elated, distraught, giddy and glum — all before she gets out of bed in the morning. She's equally unstable behind a motorized vehicle or an electric toothbrush. When the PMS spaceship lands, you're never quite sure where to recruit help...a suicide hotline or Disneyland®.

**The good news:** Things are never dull.
**The bad news:** Whiplash.

# What you can do:

While you're waiting for her circus to leave town, you've got two choices: Get a tub of popcorn and watch the daily PMS performances or make like a disappearing act and vanish!

If you choose to stay, attempt to be useful by smiling, nodding, cuddling, whatever keeps Sue on steady ground and you out of the spotlight. You can play the "victim card" later in the month after the wacky winds have passed. After all, you have feelings too, and being threatened with castration monthly is starting to grate.

Tread carefully if you want to unburden yourself. Hold her hands to express sincerity – and to prevent her from slugging you. Stay away from using words such as "insane" or "certifiable" to describe her behavior during PMS. Instead, focus on how you feel: "I feel concerned when you set my Playboys® on fire" or "I'm hurt when you booby trap the house." Get the pout and hangdog eyes down, and who knows how Sue will make it up to you later in the month.

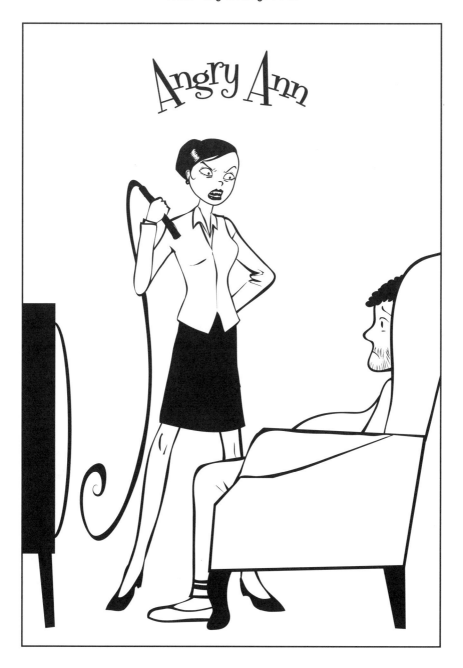

# Angry Ann (mostly "e" answers)

Angry Ann was undoubtedly a dictator of a medium-sized country in a previous life. She's more vicious than a rabid dog when she barks: "Don't wear that!" "Pick that up!" "What the hell is wrong with you?" "Do I have to do everything myself?" The only safe answer during this pre-period period is a numb and automatic, "Yes, dear!" (You often mumble these words in your sleep or when startled by a random car alarm.)

During **PMS**, this woman possesses extraordinary powers. She can see a stain on dark carpet or hear you mutter from two states away. Through cement walls or vacuum-packed seals, she can sniff out alcohol on your breath, an unfamiliar perfume or anything chocolate. Angry Ann is sometimes known by her other names: Satan, Antichrist, Ice Queen, the Wicked Witch of the west, east, north or south.

**The good news:** She can chill your beer with her stare.
**The bad news:** She carries mace – and your testicles – on her keychain.

# What you can do:

Never ask Angry Ann leading questions like "What can I do to help?" or you're likely to hear "Drop dead!" Instead, disarm her with affection: "You're scary, but I adore you" or "Eye-bulging is a complete turn-on." We don't recommend any physical contact, however, especially when she's holding a curling iron, casserole or vibrator.

As lethal as Ann can be, try to remember that she feels powerless over PMS and no matter what she calls you, don't take it personally. Believe it or not, every time she nails you for some screw-up, real or imagined, she feels (almost) as lousy as you do; once her PMS passes, she regrets her behavior. So keep tabs. You might be able to milk this for at least one "get out of mowing the lawn" pass.

Make an effort to please her. Bring her breakfast in bed or dangle something shiny in front of her – think jewelry, not a broken bottle. If she hurls any of the above back at you, try a different tack. Encourage her to vent her frustrations with shared physical activity: a walk, a pillow fight, or (should you be so lucky) sex.

# 10 Rules for Men to Live By (Literally!) During PMS

1. Give her space. Stand back – preferably in another time zone!*

2. Make **NO** comments about her appearance. It doesn't matter if her face is swollen to the size of a globe and her hair looks like there are wild creatures living in it, go rent a *Three Stooges* DVD and shut up!*

3. If she attempts to apologize for her completely irrational behavior, just nod and smile. It could be a trick.*

4. Remember at all times that it's what she meant, not what she said. Good luck with that.*

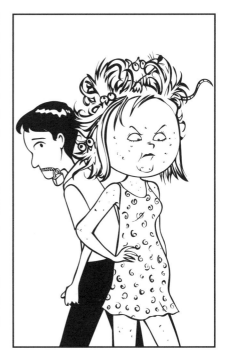

5. Silence is golden...and healthy! Tiptoe on that thin ice and avoid the cardinal sins: humming, throat-clearing, sneezing, coughing, belching, farting, chewing, sighing, slurping, crunching, tapping, snoring and finally, breathing.*

6. Never refuse to buy her feminine products. It's a good excuse to **GET OUT OF THE HOUSE.** Or, stock up and hide supplies in the garage – you'll avoid embarrassing check-out lines and she'll still think you're out. Invest in a well-stocked mini-fridge, and you've bought time alone with a cold beverage.*

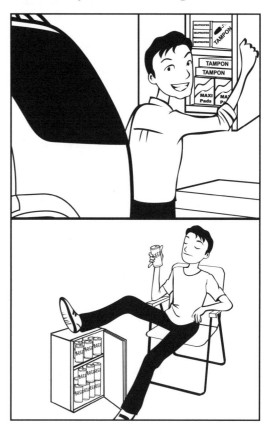

7. Don't offer sympathy. Do offer sympathy. Be forewarned that the wrong choice at the wrong time will require you to **DUCK! ***

8. Rehearse excuses why you can't wear the shirt she bought you with the bulls-eye on it. We're hoping this one's fairly obvious.*

9. Keep the following within arm's reach: a heating pad, an ice pack, ibuprofen, a good merlot, chocolate with nuts, chocolate without nuts, holy water and the number for the local crisis hotline – for you.*

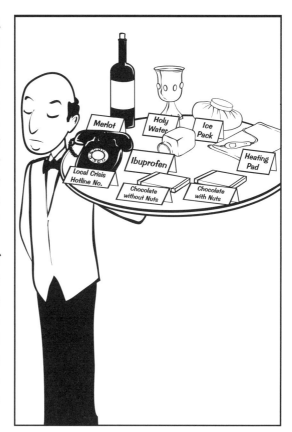

10. Familiarize yourself with the signs that the cyclical cyclone is approaching. Hide all motorized machinery, sharp utensils and reflective surfaces accordingly.*

*   *Realize that rules change and all bets are off during **PMS**. Be ready to shift gears faster than a **NASCAR**® driver because her hormones can take you on the ride of your life!*

# Just the Facts, Man

Why all the fuss? you ask. Men have hormones, too! Remember the Clearasil® years? The nocturnal emissions? The beer-goggle blurs? Your hormonal woes may have lasted through your teens or early 20s, but women have to put up with them from their first periods through menopause.

If you're like most men, PMS is about as interesting as bargain hunting for linens; however, there are facts that you need to know to protect yourself against the dragon lady wearing your loved one's clothes. Plus, you'll have the added bonus of seeming well-informed and sensitive should the subject come up over beernuts at poker night. (Yeah, right.)

Here's what you've been dying to ask, but not willing to die asking:

Q: **Is PMS for real or does it belong in the fake-orgasm-I-have-a-headache category of women's behavior?**

A: PMS isn't an urban legend, an excuse, or a life-sentence of misery – for either of you. About half of all women experience PMS at some point in their lives. Really.

Q: What causes the women in my life to turn crazier than Mike Tyson?

A: PMS is caused by hormonal changes during the menstrual cycle but can be aggravated by diet, childbirth, stress, you, switching birth control pills, lack of exercise, vitamin or mineral deficiencies and you.

Q: Zits, migraines, backaches, hissy fits...what's next, boils and chin hair?

A: Unfortunately, there are more than 150 identified symptoms of PMS, both physical and emotional, ranging from migraines and bloating to anxiety and plate throwing. (For more about symptoms, check out "Ms. Jekyll and You Better Hide!" on page 27 in the other half of this book.)

Q: My mom wasn't like this, how come my girlfriend/wife is?

A: Don't go there. Nothing good can come from comparing your mother to a woman you're sleeping with.

Q: Alright, but she wasn't always like this. Was she hiding it?

A: Symptoms can start with a woman's first period or may begin later in life. PMS can be triggered by countless reasons that are being researched by male scientists as desperate as you.

$Q$: **When will the misery end?**

$A$: The only known cure for PMS is menopause (another hell, another book) and that comes with a truckload of its own sweaty symptoms. Although there's no cure, many women are able to eliminate most of their symptoms with lifestyle changes.

$Q$: **During PMS, my sister lives on Tylenol® and my wife has a twice-a-day Baskin-Robbins® habit. How come they're different?**

$A$: Every woman experiences PMS differently, though they all seem equally pissed off.

$Q$: **Is she looking for sympathy?**

$A$: Are you looking for sex?

$Q$: **How do I know if it's PMS or something else...like rabies?**

$A$: The worst symptoms usually occur two to 10 days before a woman's period then disappear completely when her period begins. Women who are cranky all month long do not have PMS, they're just evil; what characterizes symptoms as PMS-related is their timing.

$Q$: **Will I ever get laid again?**

$A$: PMS can affect a woman's sex drive. Usually, it makes you seem about as attractive as a garden gnome. In turn, premenstrual bingeing, bloating, and crazed outbursts make women feel about as attractive as you look to them.

Q: **Does PMS really affect breast size? Sounds promising.**

A: Breast-swelling is not as appealing to women as it is to men. Refer to the previous question and answer.

Q: **Should she see a doctor (or an exorcist)?**

A: Women with serious PMS that interferes with their daily lives need to seek medical help.

Q: **Is it my fault? During PMS, everything seems to be my fault.**

A: Contrary to what she may scream, PMS isn't anyone's fault. Not yours, not your wife's, sister's, girlfriend's, coworker's, etc. That said, you are in charge of how you to respond to the crying jags and discomfort that the women in your life experience – just as they are responsible for taking steps to overcome their PMS.

# Bone Up, Boys!

In the other side of this book, women can find everything they need to know to get rid of their symptoms and beat their hormones into submission. For extra credit, feel free to check out "their side" to help the woman you love with her recovery plan.

On the other hand, if you're a bottom-line kind of guy and don't want to examine every detail of her recovery, here are the money shots:

* First, she needs to track her symptoms to diagnose and treat her PMS. She might find out that it's not PMS – in which case this book will make a lovely paper weight.

✳ A low-fat diet and plenty of exercise will help. You might want to try it, too, before you hit middle-age and your belly needs its own zip code.

✳ Alcohol and caffeine make PMS worse. For her, not for you.

✳ Vitamin and mineral supplements, especially calcium, magnesium and B6 can kick serious PMS ass. Herbal remedies work, and there a few that can jump-start a woman's sex drive (see pages 72-73 on the women's side). Do we have your attention?

✳ Give her some quiet time to help with stress reduction – hers and yours.

✳ Unless you have a flak jacket and industrial-strength jock, don't try to talk about her issues during PMS. After her period, when she's symptom-free, ask her what you can do to help.

✳ Give her a copy of this book if she doesn't have one already. Same goes for your coworkers, co-ed softball league gal pals, and anyone else with breasts who's been acting stranger than usual. Be sure to stay out of arm's reach, smile broadly and say, "I thought you'd find this funny" rather than "Your moods are creeping me out and I'm terrified of you."

If you still want to know more about the road to PMS independence, flip to the other side of this book and read on. If not, good luck and God bless.

# Things a Man Should NEVER Say During PMS

**"WHAT'S WRONG?"**

✳ You'll only make this mistake once.

**"HOW ARE YOU FEELING?"**

✳ Isn't it obvious from the swollen, contorted heap of flesh moaning on the couch?

**"GOOD MORNING!"**

✳ Nothing is good.

**"ARE YOU EXPECTING YOUR 'SPECIAL FRIEND'?"**

✳ Avoid nicknames ("code red," "monthly visitor," "Aunt Flo," etc.) women use for their impending periods. Unless you have ovaries of your own, steer clear.

**"I UNDERSTAND."**

✳ You don't.

## "YOU LOOK FINE."

✳ She knows she doesn't, so you're better off choking on your saliva or feigning a heart attack if she asks about her appearance.

## "IT MUST BE THAT TIME OF THE MONTH."

✳ It may be clear to you after she's flung the sixth pair of jeans that won't zip across the room, or starts to bawl when a contestant misses the Double Jeopardy!® question, but you're the last person she wants pointing it out!

## "PASS THE SALT (PEPPER, KETCHUP, WHATEVER)."

✳ Eat your food bland or get it yourself. Chasing condiments is better than dodging them.

## "WHAT'S FOR BREAKFAST (LUNCH, DINNER)?"

✳ Get real.

## "WE'RE OUT OF CHOCOLATE."

✳ Maintain several stashes or endure the wrath of Attila the Hungry.

## "A WOMAN'S BODY IS A MIRACLE."

✳ This may seem like safe territory, but after hemorrhaging monthly since the age of 11, she's over the miraculous part.

**"YOU'RE SO CUTE WHEN YOU MAKE THAT ANGRY FACE."**

✳ This is not reverse psychology – it's suicide!

**"I'M GOING OUT WITH THE GUYS TO GIVE YOU SOME SPACE."**

✳ Firstly, she thinks all your friends are idiots. Secondly, she wants you to suffer, too.

**"STOP KIDDING AROUND. WE BOTH KNOW THAT GUN ISN'T LOADED."**

✳ Enough said.

# The PMS Protection Plan

We know that a woman with **PMS** is scarier than seeing your mother naked, but you don't have to change your address to protect yourself. Instead, there are techniques you can use to survive the temporary madness while your Premenstrual Princess hog-ties her hormones.

Face it: There are things you do that aggravate her and her **PMS**. They may be the same slip-ups that for the rest of the month would result only in "the look" or a door slam, but during **PMS** coudl provoke a nuclear meltdown. Whether it's forgetting she likes her kung pao chicken extra spicy or lingering too long on a *Baywatch* rerun as you channel surf, there are certain triggers in every relationship. But, set off a premenstrual woman, and she'll be on your ass faster than Siegfried & Roy.

Think of the following coping strategy as a **PMS** insurance policy. It covers your butt while she makes the necessary repairs.

## Stop, Drop and Roll

Forgive us for stating the obvious, but we're men. Men rebuild carburetors, invade countries, go commando! And, we avoid couple's counseling at all costs. So before you find yourself calculating alimony, try our **PMS** Protection Plan.

It's a new twist on the Stop, Drop & Roll of fire safety. It may not save you from a burning building, but it could save you from burning one down!

Here's how it works:

First, STOP those irritating habits that drive her nuts, or at least cut back. Make a list if you have to: 1) Take better aim at the laundry hamper; 2) Stop leaving the empty juice carton in the fridge; 3) Don't scratch the family jewels while she's around; and 4) Stop calling your penis pet names (unless she made them up). This is just a sample list, but we have faith that you can come up with your own. Whatever it is that you do to send hormonal bullets flying like it's Friday night in Baghdad, STOP doing it. Replace those life-threatening behaviors with life-saving ones like bringing her a dozen Harlequin Romance® novels (which will keep her away from other family members) or any other peace offerings.

Next, DROP the notion that she can just stop "acting" this way. She's not acting. Of course, she'd rather be the woman of your dreams, but accept that she might be a nightmare until she puts her own PMS strategies into action. While you're at it, DROP any thoughts of reasoning with her while she's mid-rant. It won't work and if there are power tools nearby, things could get really messy.

Finally, you need to ROLL. That means letting go, as in "roll with the PMS punches." We know it will be difficult, but you have to accept that a woman (or many women) in your life have PMS,

and changing your identity through radical cosmetic surgery isn't a viable option. It doesn't mean roll over and play dead. It does mean be supportive. Instead of wondering why she goes ape month after month, encourage her to do something to stop the cycle. Be her hormone hero!

# Woman Speak

"That's not what you said!" "How am I supposed to know that's what you meant? I'm not a mind reader!" Since the beginning of time, men will be the first to admit they stink at reading between the lines. What they see – and hear – is what they count on getting. The trouble with that is women have a language all their own, which they expect men to understand by osmosis.

Unless you're psychic, try brushing up on the following translations. Keep this list handy the next time your lady love has something on her mind that she expects you to read.

| When she says: | She really means: |
| --- | --- |
| Maybe. | NO! |
| I'll think about it. | Not a chance in hell. |
| We need... | I want... |
| That's interesting. | Are you still speaking? |
| Does my butt look big? | Tell me I'm hot. |
| Sure, go ahead. | Watch your back. |

| When she says: | She really means: |
|---|---|
| Are you wearing that? | You've got to be kidding! |
| I'll be ready in a minute. | You have time to make a sandwich, watch Sports Center® and take a crap. |
| Pizza's fine. | Cheap jerk. |
| I need some time to process everything. | I want you to twist in the wind while I decide how you're going to pay. |
| I missed you. | The trash has to go out. |
| Fine. | Oh, it's SO not fine! |
| I'm not mad. | Of course I'm mad, you baboon! |
| We need to communicate better. | Agree with me. |
| Whatever. | &#@! YOU! |

# PMS Alert

When everything you say is wrong, the kids are hiding under the couch, the dog has moved in with the neighbors and your partner is practically unrecognizable, it might be time to check the calendar.

Thing is, while you're busy plotting world domination, or at least how to win the office NFL® pool, you don't have time to keep track of her hormones. Instead, use a service like **PMS Red Flag** (www.pmsredflag.com) that will notify you on the first day or every day of the monthly siege. Think of it like a distress signal warning you of impending doom. Getting a **PMS Alert** by email will help you make your way to the bomb shelter (the nearest bar or golf course) without sustaining any injuries.

**PMS Red Flag** can also help you to avoid scheduling family vacations or any other anticipated events during her worst days. Or, use the pmsredflag.com year-at-a-glance calendar to know when to send her on a trip with a girlfriend or surprise her with an airline ticket to...anywhere. You can also plan for some relief by working out in the evening; odds are good you won't see her at the gym during **PMS**.

If PMS follows you to the office where female coworkers all seem to be going nuts at the same time, remember that women who work or live together frequently have simultaneous menstrual cycles. Use the email reminders to give you a head's up so you can keep your head down when PMS does its business at yours.

If you've been doing your best but need a break, take advantage of the advance warning by scheduling a business trip, a boy's weekend or an overdue visit with distant relatives (preferably ones she doesn't like) around her premenstrual misery. There's a reason some men swear that PMS stands for Pass My Suitcase.

## Run, Forrest, Run

Once you know when PMS is darkening your doorstep, check out other tried and true avoidance/survival techniques:

* If you're not into fishing or camping — or any other activity that she would never do — now's the time to start!

* Put in some extra hours at the office to minimize your exposure time. If she complains, remind her it's so you can both enjoy the benefits of your six-figure income later on.

* Turn off your cell phone.

* If you are playing the field, try to date women on different cycles so you have more options during the month.

* If your boss has PMS, try to do your "fieldwork" during this time.

* Attend a weekend workshop. Reminder: "It's for our future, honey!"

* Take her to a concert or movie. Others in the audience will prevent her from talking to you.

# Once in a Blue...PMS

Did you know a woman can have two PMS episodes in one month? Women, on average, get their period every 28 days. Let's say your beloved gets her period on the 3rd of January and the 31st of January. That means you should be prepared for a double whammy of PMS, with symptoms occurring before both periods. How lucky can one guy get?

# PMS Got Your Tongue?
## Avoiding the Mouth Traps

Dying to cut the chit-chat and the crap? Does everything you say increase the odds of you sleeping on the couch? Next month, stop disastrous, can't-win conversations with one-line replies – and a speedy exit! Sure, some of the following responses require Academy Award® winning performances from you, but it'll be worth it. Once you get the hang of it, you can prevent the game known as "your life" being called on account of PMS.

| She Says: | You Say: |
|---|---|
| I look like a stripper with these swollen boobs! | Would you like a hug? |
| I want a divorce. | Let's go shopping! |
| If you ate the last jelly donut, you're a dead man. | Did you lose weight? |
| You stink. | You smell great! |
| Do you know of a lethal poison that won't show up in an autopsy? | Let me take you out to dinner tonight so you don't have to cook. |

| She Says: | You Say: |
|---|---|
| My fat clothes are tight!... (sob! snivel! snot!) ...Call me "Shamu!" | I love you! ("Come to Papa Whale" is the express route to the PMS doghouse.) |
| Were you always this short? | I apologize. |
| Do you love me?/Life sucks/Let's adopt a child from another country/I'm leaving you for your brother and we're booked on Jerry Springer. | Yes, dear. (Bonus: This versatile, PMS-proof answer doesn't require you to actually hear what she said first.) |

# Gifts That Keep on Giving

In addition to watching your words, minding your manners and updating your living will, try winning her over with gestures that show you care. Below, you'll find gold star strategies for surviving PMS that will repay you with peace and quiet:

* If she'll let you touch her, offer her a no-strings-attached massage. Convince her you want nothing in return.

* Suggest taking the kids out so she can stay home and relax ("stay home" being the key phrase here).

* Keep spa gift certificates on hand and use the element of surprise to your advantage.

* You can't go wrong with flowers or chocolate. Try both on peak PMS days.

* Offer to do the dishes and even if it's the crack of dawn, head immediately to the kitchen.

* Set up her bath with candles and a glass of wine. This should buy you an hour or so of TV.

* Sign up for a massage class together. It's fun and there will be women moaning.

* Offer to fix things around the house, which will get you a gold star and some time by yourself.

# A Note From Our Relationship Coaches

In the following chapter, you'll find some valuable relationship coaching that will help you deal with your loved or not-so-loved one suffering from PMS.

Sure you can live in denial, take monthly fishing trips, pray for well-timed business travel, but whether it's at work or in your personal life, sooner or later you'll have to take it like a man. That means confronting the PMS mess and learning how to love your princess back to health. Read on and you'll discover how.

—Elizabeth Goodman & Herb Tanzer

# Staying Sane

Women with PMS run through a laundry list of culprits during their reproductive years: clueless parents, insensitive gynecologists, demanding bosses, and you. Man or woman, it's easier to assign blame than to fix problems. But PMS is a fact of life. It is real and it is mediated by hormones. You can't choose whether your wife, girlfriend or coworker has PMS *but* you can choose *what kind of guy you're going to be* with her PMS.

If you want to be *the good guy*, you'll have to decide whether it's more important to you to be right or to be happy. We all know someone who is hell bent on being right. He's the one who'll stick to his guns no matter what logic he's confronted with; she's the one who'll argue 'til she's blue in the face to prove her point. These people are seldom well-liked and, in spite of "being right," they're usually not happy.

Most couples have the same fight over and over again. It may assume different forms, but it's ultimately about each person's "rightness," whether it's the best route to the mall or whose turn it is to do household chores. Over time, we tend to get "dug in" or stuck with that rightness. We're so sure we don't like X, don't want to try Y, can't change Z, that there's no possibility for anything else.

If you're convinced that PMS is all in her head, you're not going to accept that a massage and a little compassion could change your relationship for the better. Similarly, if she's committed to the notion that she's stuck with PMS, she's probably not going to stop eating the refined sugar and fried everything that fuels the unhappy cycle. Allowing that there are alternative ways to think about PMS, and life's other challenges, opens a world of possibilities and hope. It's all about giving in a little to get back a lot!

# Positively PMS

Fact: If someone says "don't think about breasts" you're mentally flipping through Playboy® before you know it. It's an automatic male response. Similarly, you experience automatic responses to situations in your relationship. If, for instance, your wife or girlfriend forgets something on the grocery list, is there a broken record of "She never remembers the beer! She always forgets the things I want" running endlessly in your head? Now ask yourself, *Do these thoughts help or hurt your relationship?* Are you focused on the positive or the negative? If the answer is that you're focused on the negative, what alternative thoughts might make you – and your Premenstrual Princess – feel better?

What you think determines how you feel: Go to work with an "I have to be here" attitude instead of "I am lucky I get to be here!" and your days will be endless. Similarly, if you sit down for a heart-to-heart with your wife or girlfriend with a lousy attitude, the outcome will be same – lousy. If you aren't thinking positively about dealing with her PMS, she's the only one

who'll make progress. And where does that leave you exactly? Better get with her PMS program, don't you think?

# Fight "Fight or Flight"

Neuroscientists at the Universities of Wisconsin and Virginia recently completed a study on a husband's touch. The results showed that women under extreme stress felt immediate relief at the touch of their husbands' hands. "Great!" you say, "Now where's my relief?" In case you're a beer short of a six pack, we'll spell it out: When she feels better, you both feel better!

The energy that courses through women when they're mid-PMS is like lightning – lethal if it hits you head on. Believe it or not, hugging that same woman focuses her tension so it can dissipate; touching her releases that deadly energy, alleviating some of the symptoms just like a lightning rod conducts millions of volts back into the earth.

Of course, the last thing you want to do is snuggle up with the source of your suffering. You're more likely to rethink gun control than imagine that a hug could change the course of the premenstrual tide. We recognize it'll take every ounce of self-control and discipline to move in the direction of the problem, but the only way out is to get *connected* – by touch or a kind word. As bad as you feel, she feels worse. For you to be responsive (emotionally and physically) is a real breakthrough in intimacy that can improve your relationship long after a bad bout of PMS is forgotten.

# In Her Shoes

Ask her to be honest about PMS (after the worst has passed) and pay attention when she talks. Ignoring her hormones is like

denying that you're in danger. Chances are everyone's going to get hurt. It can be as simple as asking, "Honey, what do you need from me?" and then really listening...with the TV OFF, not just muted.

Put yourself in her pumps, metaphorically, for a moment. When she has PMS, do you think a woman feels particularly loved or lovable? Help change that attitude by telling her that you love her and that she's beautiful. Let go of thoughts like, "Well, she knows I love her. I'm here aren't I?" That's how guys think, not women.

Here's how the rest of that conversation goes: You might say, "Why do I have to keep telling you I love you?" She says, "You haven't told me lately!" You remind her, "I told you 10 minutes ago." She snaps, "That ain't lately!" and, during PMS, it's true.

Changing the automatic responses will change the direction of the downhill dialogue and ultimately, the course of the monkey wrench PMS can throw into any relationship. Oh, and don't think for one moment that we aren't giving her the same advice, because we are. You'll both need to pitch in to free yourselves from the mayhem.

# The Finish Line: Being Happy

When all else is said and done, here's a good rule of thumb to remember: *Whoever gets sane first takes care of the other one.* In all likelihood, until she has her PMS licked, you're going to be first to reach the finish line.

As you begin to battle about something minor, rather than engaging "the enemy," keep in mind that this is a volatile time and

56

before you know it, a spat can turn into divorce court testimony. Disengage. That doesn't mean being distant or silent, but if you're arguing over where to park or what to have for dinner, give in! It's a great way to restore a little peace and what did it really cost you? It comes back to the notion of whether it's more important to you to be right or to be happy. Remember, happy involves sex.

# About the Authors

## Brian Young

For nearly four decades, Mr. Young didn't know if it was him or PMS when the women in his life acted in a way that he considered to be a little crazy...okay, sometimes a lot crazy. Through years of research and "field work" as a serial dater, he asked his life coach, Herb Tanzer, this question: "What's the deal with women and PMS?!" After discussing the realities of PMS symptoms and providing a different viewpoint to consider, Mr. Tanzer encouraged Mr. Young to channel his frustrations toward promoting discussion with women and men and formulate successful strategies to help both genders better cope with the effects. Soon, *The Prince and the PMS* was born.

Mr. Young is a successful real estate entrepreneur who lives in San Diego, California. He is currently in a long-term relationship – a fact that he credits to the tips outlined in this book. Contact him at Brian@PMSCentral.com.

# Herb Tanzer

Since the 1980s, Herb Tanzer has been a sought-after personal and professional life coach, designing and delivering workshops and seminars that empower individuals in communication, teamwork, partnership and entrepreneurial endeavors. Mr. Tanzer, along with co-author and wife Elizabeth Goodman, provides men with vital insight about the impact PMS can have on relationships and suggests how to utilize male gender traits to communicate compassion.

Known as an experienced and honored contributor in life coaching circles, Mr. Tanzer has hosted his own television show on CNN and subsequently worked with the NBC and ABC networks.  He graduated with honors from Cornell University and is a published author and sought-after speaker.  He and Ms. Goodman live in North San Diego County.  Contact him at Herb@PMSCentral.com.

# Lori Shaw-Cohen

Lori Shaw-Cohen is a best-selling author, editor and nationally published journalist, whose work has appeared in numerous publications for almost three decades. Formerly the Managing Editor of 'TEEN Magazine, Ms. Shaw-Cohen's parenting articles and columns, "The Parent Zone" and "Mom Central," have been featured regularly in major newspapers and regional magazines. She has appeared on television and radio, and has spoken at writers' conferences throughout the United States.

In 2005, Ms. Shaw-Cohen co-authored the national bestseller *Home Buying by the Experts*, a book for first-time homeowners. Originally from Southern California (by way of Manhattan), she moved to the Nashville area in 1996 with her husband and three children.  Contact her at LoriShawCohen@aol.com.

# Tracy Stevens

Tracy Stevens is an author, editor and book designer. After earning a degree in Writing, Literature and Publishing from Emerson College in 1993, she began work as an editorial assistant in New York. She became the Editorial Director of Quigley Publishing Company in 1997.

Ms. Stevens is a consultant to numerous publishers and authors and has ghostwritten and designed several bestselling books. In addition to her work in the publishing industry, she serves as the executive director of The Hospital to Home Foundation and has worked with other nonprofits worldwide. She has lived in Europe and the Middle East and currently resides in San Diego, California. Contact her at tracy@wordwit.com.

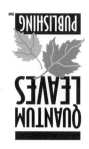

QUANTUM LEAVES
PUBLISHING SM

# The Princess and the PMS

ISBN-10: 0-9761526-1-4
ISBN-13: 978-0-9761526-1-3

First Edition. Printed in the United States of America.

BOOK DESIGN by TRACY STEVENS
CARTOONS by TURONNY FUAD/www.poggiwoggi.com
COVER ILLUSTRATIONS©CHUCK GONZALES/www.artscounselinc.com
COVER DESIGN by JOHN COSTA, New Orleans

Published by Quantum Leaves Publishing℠
Del Mar, California.
www.theprincessandthepms.com
www.quantumleaves.com

see page 168 for credits

# With thanks to:

Jessica for the support and encouragement,
Audrey and David McKnight for their artistic skills and Ellen
Stiefler for keeping us on the right legal path

Tilak for helping us to be mindful

Bob, Joshua, Drew and Logan, the home team, for all the
laughter, light and love along the way

Mom, Ava, Splinky and Charger for
their boundless love and support

# Our Lawyers Made Us Say This...

# A Note to Our Princesses

Have you turned into one of those women you can't stand? You know the type, wound so tight that if they ever removed the stick from their behinds they'd fly off to another hemisphere – snarling and snapping commands at loved ones or sobbing over a broken nail, hot-tempered and stone-cold scary during certain days – or weeks – of the month.

So, you've got PMS. Join the club, or better yet, DON'T! Premenstrual syndrome has been the bane of women (and men) since Cleopatra, who was rumored to be barge-bound for days before she laid waste to an empire. Month after month in boardrooms and bedrooms, carpools and classrooms, PMS wreaks havoc on otherwise happy lives. PMS is an equal opportunity menace, without regard for race, creed or class, turning countless productive, well-balanced women into eye-bulging, frying pan-wielding cartoon characters.

No matter how we try, husbands, lovers, children and colleagues are bound to get hit by (not always) stray hormonal buckshot. We drag our symptoms to work with us, on the errands we run and at the end of the day, find ourselves in an unwelcome threesome with PMS and our significant other. What's worse, after our period arrives and our cyclical nemesis departs, it seems like only a few "normal" days pass before we're facing yet another round of PMS. And men wonder why we're pissed off.

In the following pages, instead of getting knocked out month after month, you'll discover how to fight back when PMS coldcocks your world. We'll help you to identify and track your symptoms so you have a better description than "I want to die" for what ails you (see "Ms. Jekyll and You Better Hide!" on page 27). You'll learn different ways to treat symptoms that include getting your calcium from foods other than ice cream and using supplements and herbs for everything from migraines to a hard-core Ding Dong® addiction. We'll encourage you to heal like a princess in "PMS: A License to Chill" and show you how to make it work at work in spite of your PMS in "On the Job With PMS: Don't Get Worked Up." There are even special bonus chapters, "The 'I' of the Storm" and "Getting Well, Together" with advice from relationship experts who have a unique way of handing PMS its walking papers.

The toll that PMS can take on relationships doesn't have to be permanent. Collateral damage can be repaired by employing new and improved communication skills — that don't involve firearms — with those you love (see "Love Me Tender...and Bloated" on page 77). Speaking of the bonds that tie (and sometimes strangle) you might have noticed that only half of this book is for you. *The Prince and the PMS* on the flip side is written and designed for the men in your life. Yes, there are a few "on the rag" jokes and lots of pictures to hold their attention, but there's also plenty of practical information about PMS so they'll stop asking stupid questions like, "Isn't there a pill or something you can take?" We suggest you give this book to someone you love...gently.

Our approach to managing and ultimately breaking free from PMS is for real women like you who have relationships, jobs, kids, late-night food benders, bathtubs with rings and a genuine desire to put PMS behind them. In the process, we hope you'll find some humor, too. Laughter can be great therapy, and between us women, let's admit there's plenty of PMS fodder for the funny mill, even if we don't quite see it that way until our symptoms have passed!

So, kick off your shoes, put up your swollen tootsies, and prepare to deal with your not-so-inner Premenstrual Princess. Hope and help are on the way! Read on to see how you can evict her highness from your castle – while keeping the king and the tiara – and reign supreme over your PMS-free forever after.

# Contents

# Who Are You?

Have you ever found yourself wondering, "Who said that?" after a surprisingly familiar voice (your own!) barked ultimatums at a loved one or bit the head off the cable repair guy? Did you ever freak out over burnt toast? Wolf down a double cheeseburger and then remember you're a vegetarian?

Blubbering over a snagged stocking may be a telltale sign you have **PMS**, but do you know what type of **PMS** has sidetracked your sanity? Take the following quiz to find out if you're masquerading monthly as Attila the Hungry, Scary Poppins, Weeping Beauty or another premenstrual character.

1.  **During "that time of month," what sets you off?**

    a.  people referring to it as "that time of month"
    b.  the "damn dryer" shrinking all your clothes
    c.  Victoria's Secret® catalogs
    d.  the male species
    e.  daylight

2.  **Your worst symptoms include:**

    a.  retaining more water than the Hoover Dam
    b.  chugging maple syrup
    c.  sprouting pimples like a 14-year-old boy
    d.  replacing family photos with the ones that came with the frames
    e.  insisting people address you as "Empress"

### 3. You find comfort in:

a. sleeping from Friday evening to Monday morning
b. anything mashed, smothered or dipped in chocolate
c. blasting Pearl Jam and smashing furniture
d. flipping the bird instead of saying "hello"
e. disseminating creepy urban legends

### 4. On your most difficult days, you wish your man would:

a. show a little sympathy
b. buy a Dairy Queen®
c. morph into Jude Law
d. move
e. grow a uterus and suffer, too

### 5. Right before your period, your sex drive is:

a. Pardon me?
b. Is this a trick question?
c. That's not funny.
d. Ha! Ha! Ha! Ha!
e. all of the above.

### 6. While PMSing, which wisecrack would you most likely use?

a. "Nice cologne. Have you been marinating in it?"
b. "Well, this day was a waste of clean sweats!"
c. "How many times do I have to flush before you go away?"
d. "You say I'm a bitch like it's a bad thing."
e. "SSSShhhh. I'm trying to imagine you with a personality."

### 7. When PMS passes, you...

a. remember nothing
b. pretend to remember nothing
c. spend the next two weeks apologizing
d. change your phone number
e. brush your hair

**8. Your most memorable PMS episode was when you:**

 a. made the pizza delivery man cry
 b. named your twin girls Ben and Jerry
 c. quit your job – twice in the same day
 d. changed your religion
 e. told your husband he wasn't the biological father of your kids

# Answers

Add up how many "a" answers you have, how many "b" answers, etc., and discover who inhabits your body every month. It's possible – in fact, likely – for you to exhibit more than one "personality," so be sure to read all relevant descriptions.

# Lois Pain (mostly "a" answers)

You hit the PMS lottery! Everything hurts – and you make sure everyone knows it! You pop Motrin® like M&Ms® (by the pound) and for a few days every month you wear nothing but a heating pad and a scowl. When loved ones suggest exercise and fresh air, you walk briskly to the door and show them out! Frequent urination has forced you to put a mailbox and a George Foreman® Grill in the master bath. And, how 'bout a little vinegar with that oil? Your complexion is so greasy the only thing that keeps your glasses from sliding off is the giant zit on your nose.

# Attila the Hungry (mostly "b" answers)

For you, God can be found in a glazed donut. You'd sell your soul for another slice of pie. Hell, you'd sell your kids for more chocolate pudding. The Tasmanian Devil has nothing on you. Whirring around the kitchen like a tornado with a mouth, you chomp through slabs of barbeque beef or piles of brownies like a

chainsaw. You're a salivating, mayonnaise-gulping, ravenous madwoman, who'd stab anyone reaching for the last piece of bacon. The neighborhood all-you-can-eat buffet has barred you for life. The rest of the month is spent nibbling a lettuce leaf and some cottage cheese to make up for the beast's binge.

# Scary Poppins (mostly "c" answers)

A spoonful of sugar helps the mood stabilizers go down. Also known as Miss Wiggy, your premenstrual persona contemplates the meaning of life one moment and the next, is enraged over the preempting of a soap opera. Family members have suggested nametags for your different personalities. Trying to keep up with your fickle feelings during PMS is like watching ping pong champions on speed. Planning anything – a wedding, oil change or a bikini wax – should probably be avoided during this time.

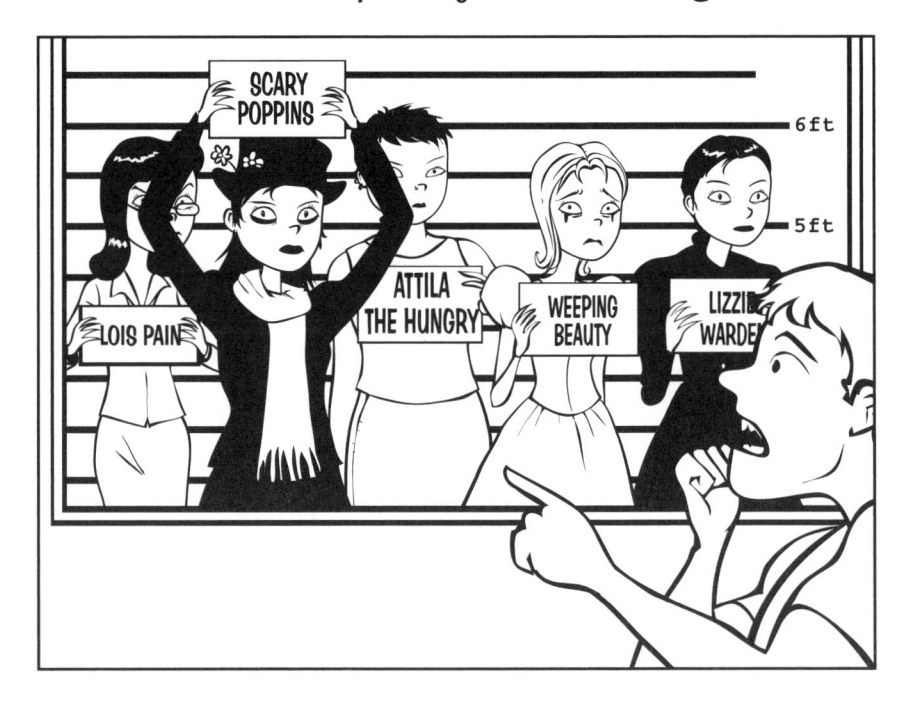

# Weeping Beauty (mostly "d" answers)

For a few days every month, you leave a puddle everywhere you go. Because the clubbing of baby seals and running out of hair product provoke the same flood of tears, relatives are clueless what to do to help – other than follow you around with a sponge and Visine®. During your visit to this PMS fun zone, referring to you as overly sensitive is an understatement. Since anything from Nora Jones to Marilyn Manson CDs can trigger a torrent, it's wise to pass up a soundtrack to your suffering. Although you've learned to do numerous tasks while the face faucets are stuck on full blast, calligraphy and candle lighting are a bitch.

# Lizzie Warden (mostly "e" answers)

Prisoners of the hell you inflict would find Alcatraz more comfortable. After all, if you're suffering, why shouldn't everyone else suffer, too? Is a little revenge really such a bad thing? Sarcasm is another service you offer. Your husband suggests you get a part-time job, and you respond, "I already work very hard at making your life miserable!" The bumper sticker on your car reads: How's My Driving? Call 1-800 KISS MY ASS. Until PMS passes, nothing is right: the house needs painting, your car's too old, the dog is ugly, the neighbors are Nazis.

*"Women complain about PMS, but I think of it as the only time of the month when I can be myself."* —Roseanne Barr

# Say Hello to My Little Friend...PMS

Most of the U.S. male population has a notion that a woman shouldn't occupy the Oval Office in case a particularly nasty bout of PMS ends in nuclear holocaust. On the other hand, if a woman were elected president, her efforts would be focused on finding a cure for PMS. Women know that's the most direct route to obtaining world peace!

## The More, the Miserable

Look to your right. Now look to your left. Chances are a suffering sister is sitting beside you — especially if you happen to be in your gynecologist's waiting room. Studies show that about half of all women experience PMS at some point in their lives. By any standard, that's an epidemic. Yet, scientists can't agree on the cause or a course of treatment for a syndrome with more than 150 identified symptoms that range from bloating and irritability to migraines and an inexplicable fascination with ninja movies.

7

PMS afflicts women worldwide with certain cultural similarities. For example, women in China cite an increased sensitivity to cold but rarely report a change in mood, the most common complaint of American women. There are a few lucky souls who experience positive premenstrual changes, such as bursts of energy, increased creativity and sex drive, but they remain in the minority (and the Witness Protection Program).

The bad news is that the only known cure for PMS is menopause* when cramps and tampons are exchanged for a mustache and adult diapers; the good news is that there are take-charge techniques that can minimize your symptoms and help you to cope physically and mentally with your other personality, the premenstrual monster. Hang on ladies, help is on the way!

✷ *Something to ponder, preferably when you're not experiencing PMS: What do the following conditions have in common? PreMENstrual, MENopause, MENtal illness. And why isn't it called a HERsterectomy? Hmmm....*

## Real Women Wear White

Contrary to what some boneheads think, PMS is as real as jock itch and about as fun. But, like jock itch, although inconvenient and highly annoying, PMS isn't a disease or a reason to be ostracized from the human race. You may be in excellent physical and mental health and feel quite normal for most of the month, only to experience significant physical and psychological changes during the dreaded pre-period period. Overcoming PMS is mostly about conquering biology with behavior. Like any good general marshalling her troops or successful dominatrix worth her weight in leather, you've got to know your enemy to beat it into submission.

Say Hello to My Little Friend...PMS

In case you weren't paying attention in high school sex ed., your menstrual cycle is controlled by hormones. They are the chemical messengers that make you weepy, wacky and wet and send marching orders to your ovaries telling them to ovulate. If the egg is unfertilized, the inner lining of your uterus will shed, causing your period to flow too freely when you're wearing white or have anywhere important to go.

During the menstrual cycle, low levels of one hormone stimulate rising levels of another, creating a pattern that repeats itself monthly. There are six hormones that control the menstrual cycle, but the ones most commonly referred to are estrogen, progesterone and testosterone. Think of them as the vanilla, chocolate and strawberry of women's hormones. (To learn more, check out "Crash Course: Hormones 101" on page 73.)

Unless you're planning to hang a shingle and purchase a pair of gynecological stirrups, the most important thing to remember is that when hormones work in harmony, you will have predictable periods — and predictable PMS. Women who menstruate normally have a cycle with four phases that add up to around 28 days of fun each month. Those four phases are:

1. **Menstrual (days 1-5)** a.k.a. "Damn! I forgot to buy tampons!"
2. **Follicular (days 6-12)** a.k.a. "Thank goodness that's over!"
3. **Ovulatory (days 13-15)** a.k.a. "Here we go again!"
4. **Luteal (days 16-28)** a.k.a. "Get out of the house!"

It's during the luteal phase, when progesterone levels are low and estrogen dominates, that most women experience their worst symptoms and empathize with disgruntled postal workers.

# Timing Is Everything

*My doctor said, "I've got good news and I've got bad news. The good news is you don't have PMS. The bad news is you're a bitch."*

The best medical definition of PMS is provided by Dr. Katharina Dalton and Dr. Graham Greene, who coined the term in the 1950s: *Premenstrual Syndrome is the recurrence of symptoms before menstruation with complete absence of symptoms after menstruation.* As PMS symptoms can occur as part of other ailments, the predictable coming and going of those symptoms is the key. For example, headaches could be caused by stress, eye strain, low blood sugar or allergies; irritability could be the result of a size-2 saleswoman in the plus-size department, a slow driver in YOUR lane, your husband's 3,000th "pull my finger" request, and so on. What defines symptoms as premenstrual is their appearance *prior to* menstruation with some regularity. As with most things in life, it's all about timing. In a nutshell, if you're cranky all month, not just between ovulation and the onset of your period, you probably should be changing something other than your tampons.

Most signs of PMS can be categorized into four groups (in no particular order of misery):

**"DID YOU GET THE LICENSE PLATE OF THE TRUCK THAT HIT ME?"** These symptoms include abdominal pain and cramping, headaches, backaches, stiff neck, joint pain and muscle aches.

**"I FEEL LIKE CRAP (AND MY ASS IS THE SIZE OF MONTANA)!"** This group of symptoms includes weight gain, gas, nausea, fatigue, constipation, forgetfulness, rashes and itching.

10

## "IF IT DOESN'T RUN AWAY, I'LL EAT IT!"
Symptoms include increased appetite, cravings for sweet, fatty or salty foods, impulsive behavior and decreased concentration.

## "COME NEAR ME AND LOSE A LIMB!"
These are the most common and most difficult PMS symptoms to treat. They include anxiety, anger, nervousness, irritability, depression, low self-esteem and hypersensitivity.

You may have symptoms from each of these groups (lucky you!) or discover that your symptoms vary from month to month. Like many women, once your PMS is over, you may feign amnesia. But, you know what "they" say: Fool them once, shame on you; fool them monthly for 30 years, and you have pretty stupid family members. So, unless gullibility runs rampant in your gene pool, you'll find your symptoms are easier to treat when you have a record of exactly what they are and when they occur. To track your symptoms, use the instructions for the "Monthly 'Monstrual' Chart" on page 137. While you have PMS, this record can provide you with some clarity; once you've conquered your PMS, it will make great material for a daytime drama.

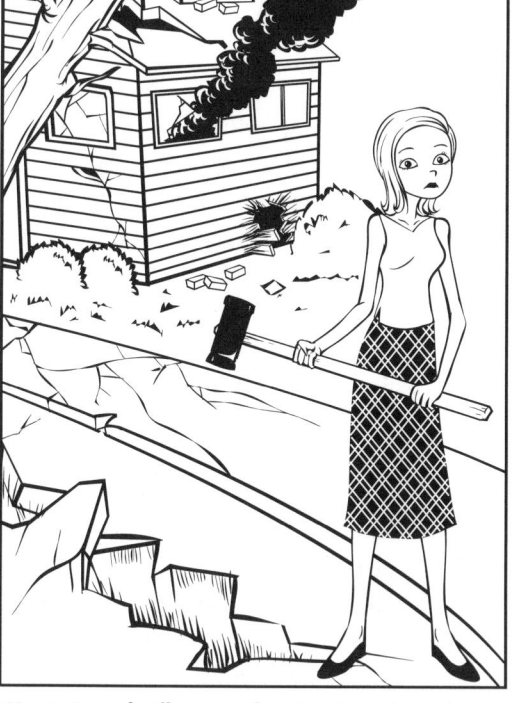

Next time, he'll remember to rinse his plate.

# Who Can We Blame?

Although it's widely accepted by the medical community that PMS is related to hormonal changes during the menstrual cycle, there is no consensus on the cause. Theories have pointed to a deficiency of progesterone, an excess of estrogen, or an imbalance between the two hormones. Others argue that low blood sugar, vitamin and mineral deficiencies or men with pinky rings and comb-overs are to blame.

Heredity appears to play a role although symptoms may differ between sisters, mothers and daughters, but feel free to blame them if you're so inclined. Researchers have also investigated the link between PMS and personality, assessing coping style, response to stress, and the level of the brain chemical serotonin (the mind's answer to chocolate).

Today, the prevailing view is that women with PMS are more sensitive to the hormonal shifts that occur during the menstrual cycle, and consequently, experience symptoms that don't affect other women (the same lucky witches, no doubt, who've been spared cellulite and blind dates with ear hair).

Of the hundreds of millions of women who have PMS, each has a different degree of sensitivity to her symptoms. Your next door neighbor may be particularly bothered by cramps and fatigue while your best friend responds more strongly to premenstrual changes in mood and wet towels on the bathroom floor. Those reactions are influenced by our lifestyle, our personalities, underlying physical or emotional issues and, in the case of the damp linens, inconsiderate family members. This presents quite a challenge to not only women trying to deal with themselves and their evil twins, but also to practitioners attempting to solve the PMS puzzle.

# Bad Attitude!

*"My license plate says 'PMS.' Nobody cuts me off."* —Wendy Liebman

We know PMS precedes our periods month after month, so why do we beat ourselves up for getting sucker-punched by the symptoms? While experts don't understand exactly what causes PMS, they do know that the walking wounded are not to blame. PMS is not triggered by your shortcomings, your weight, your career choice or even by the creepy guy in high-waters and hair gel at the office. Homemakers and CEOs, women with and without children, young and not so young, single and married, over- and underweight, heterosexual and lesbian all experience PMS.

Studies, however, have shown that there is a link between perfectionism and PMS. We gals tend to have unrealistic expectations about our own capabilities and performance. We think we can be "super moms," "have fabulous careers," practice good self-care and shoulder more than our share of the world's burdens every day while having sex like nymphomaniacs. We feel PMS should be penciled in like a doctor's appointment or PTA meeting and then condemn ourselves for succumbing to the chaos it inflicts.

## Connecting the Periods

As scientists continue to untangle the mysteries of the female body and premenstrual women continue to reach for something sweet, then salty, then sweet again, we know a couple things to be true: The amount of stress in our lives has an effect on the intensity of our PMS symptoms, and our physical and mental wellbeing impact our ability to cope with those symptoms. Throughout this book you'll see that, despite objections from loved ones several days a month, your mind and body are connected. In conquering your PMS, you'll learn to take better care of both.

A couple was at home one afternoon;
she was reading the bible while he was tidying up.

*The husband said to his wife, "You know, honey, everything you ever wanted to know about life is in here."*

*She replied, "Well, maybe not EVERYTHING, dear."*

*"Just name one thing I can't find in here," he said confidently.*

*"You won't find anything about PMS in there," she challenged.*

*He began flipping through the pages, going from one chapter to another. Finally, after several minutes, he looked up at his wife and said, "Aha! I found it! I told you everything was in here."*

*He proceeded to read, "...and Mary rode Joseph's ass...."*

# The HERstory of PMS

Women with PMS swear they can set clocks by their monthly cravings, ravings and misbehaving. Heaven help the man, or worse yet the woman, who mutters "it's all in her (rotating) head!" PMS, though not named until the 20th century, has plagued women for eons. It's as real as the uncontrollable flood of tears that follows the discovery that some inconsiderate beast ate the last two Chips Ahoy!® — even after realizing it was you — 20 minutes ago!

# Fear of Flying off the Handle

It's no accident that in the late 1990s, the scariest female pro-wrestling team in the **WWF** went by the name "PMS." In one memorable appearance, the kick-ass temptresses lured a TV announcer with come hither gestures then dealt him a swift below-the-belt blow that reduced him to a whimpering...well, wimp! PMS, now such a recognizable part of our culture that it appears everywhere from TV shows to t-shirts, is a 20th century notion. So, how did it all begin?

# A Time for Hysterics

Women's compulsion for new shoes and black slacks, not to mention the mysteries of their reproductive cycles, have always perplexed men. For thousands of years, the world's major religions have viewed menstruating women as impure, segregating them from the rest of the community, deeming them untouchable, and so on. Of course, if women had recorded history, this period might be considered as the origin of "me time."

As late as the 19th century, most of the medical community still believed that a woman's purpose in life was to reproduce with as little fuss as possible. When women complained of "female trouble" such as swelling, nervousness, insomnia, heaviness in the abdomen, muscle spasms, loss of appetite for food, or even a bad hair day, they were diagnosed with "hysteria."

Soon, any independent action by women – from belching out loud to running away with a hunky, spontaneous gold miner – was classified as hysteria. This "diagnosis" kept women out of universities and medical schools and prevented them from voting.

Said one legislator, who sounded rather "hysterical" himself, "Grant suffrage to women, and you will have to build insane asylums in every county, and establish a divorce court in every town." It was understood that women, at the mercy of their reproductive systems, weren't fit to do much of anything at all (except cook, clean, mend, wash, iron, change the toilet paper roll...but we digress.)

## Ladies, Start Your Engines

In a stroke of genius, however, a cure for hysteria was soon found. Doctors prescribed "pelvic massage" or manual stimulation of a woman's genitals to achieve "hysterical paroxysm" a.k.a. orgasm. Naturally, hysteria spread like wildfire among white, middle-class women – especially those with particularly good-looking OB-GYNs. In 1853, one doctor wrote, "I have seen young unmarried women asking every medical practitioner to institute an examination of the sexual organs." Can you blame them?

A backlash against these voracious Victorian women followed, and bed rest became the new treatment of choice. When bed rest failed, physicians beat women with wet towels or heckled and embarrassed them in front of their families and friends. However, none of that quite packed the punch of the "Big O."

## A No-Brainer

**The woman scientist who invents a vibrating tampon will make a fortune. That way we can be at our best when we're at our worst!**

By 1900, a stupendous selection of vibrating devices designed to induce orgasm and reduce hysteria was available, ranging from hand or foot-powered models to those motorized by air pressure, water turbines, gas engines and batteries. Although initially sold only to doctors, it wasn't long before American women got their hands, among other body parts, on them. In fact, the vibrator was the fifth household device to be electrified, after the sewing machine, fan, tea kettle and toaster. Apparently, it took turn-of-the-century women a few years to get their priorities straight.

Soon many low-cost models of vibrators were marketed as health and relaxation devices for home – and wagon train – use. The Swedish Vibrator Company of Chicago extolled its device as "a machine that gives 30,000 thrilling, invigorating, revitalizing penetrations per minute." In 1918, the Sears Roebuck catalog advertised vibrators that were "very satisfactory...an aid every woman appreciates." Amen to that! (For more on the benefits of orgasm, see "Choose Pleasure Over Pain" on page 109.)

Save for a few compassionate doctors with spinster patients, physicians stopped administering "help" via vibrators by the 1920s. However, hysteria, with symptoms remarkably similar to those of PMS, wasn't officially debunked by the American Psychiatric Association until 1952 (only to resurface later with the introduction of the Beatles, liposuction and Häagen-Dazs® Chocolate Chocolate Chip).

# Snap! Cackle! Freak Out!

*How many men does it take to wallpaper a PMSing woman's house? Only five if you slice them thin enough.*

A couple of decades before they killed off hysteria for good,

doctors began documenting premenstrual tension and other complaints specifically related to the menstrual cycle. In 1931, Dr. Robert T. Frank wrote about women patients who complained of being tense and irritable, crying more easily than usual, and engaging in what he termed "foolish and ill-considered actions," which, in the 1930s, may have been anything from adding potato chips to a tuna casserole to venturing out without a girdle.

As views about women changed (translation: "Maybe they're not nuts!") and research continued in earnest, it became clear that the "tension" evident during the premenstrual phase of our cycle was only part of what had to be called a "syndrome." There were too many other symptoms that constantly occurred prior to and disappeared completely with the onset of menstruation. The term Premenstrual Syndrome came from the work of two English physicians, Dr. Katharina Dalton and Dr. Raymond Greene. In 1953, they published the first paper on PMS and changed how we think about hormones and Good Housekeeping® magazine forever. (Something to ponder, ladies: Would men have ever subscribed to Good Grooming?)

It wasn't until the women's lib movement of the 1970s that PMS became firmly established in our culture and a perfectly acceptable reason to buy a submachine gun. Two sensational murder trials in the U.K. in which the courts accepted PMS as a plea of diminished responsibility paved the way. The trials received worldwide publicity, and introduced many people to PMS and the idea that premenstrual hormonal fluctuations could turn some women into both dangerous criminals and sugar-inhaling fiends. The attorney for one of the accused women said that without progesterone injections to control her PMS, the "hidden animal" in his client would again emerge to threaten society – not to mention ice cream men everywhere.

Many people believe that, "But, officer, he ate the last jellybean!" is not an excuse for irrational behavior, let alone murder, and encourages the idea that, once a month, women aren't responsible for their own actions. That may be, but let's be honest: Men have been blaming "penises with minds of their own" for their bad conduct since cavemen clubbed their first mistresses.

No matter how you feel about PMS as a defense for murder or as an excuse for keeping guacamole and chips in your glove compartment, the hoopla about hormones gave credibility to the complaints suffered by women for centuries. PMS, with its host of symptoms, became part of our culture and consciousness.

# On the Rag, Off the Christmas Card List

In the span of a few years, PMS went from unrecognized phenomenon to a label for any emotion or argument that men found annoying or insignificant. PMS lost its original medical meaning and became a slogan, and a virtual synonym for temperamental behavior. Every time a woman raised her voice or had a craving for hot fudge, a man somewhere muttered, "PMS."

PMS became a term of ridicule, trivializing our genuine anger at spouses, incompetent coworkers and Jenny Craig® commercials. Take for instance, Dr. Edgar Berman, a member of the 1970 Democratic Party Committee on National Priorities, who was quoted as saying, "Women are unfit for executive office because of raging hormonal influences." In the 21st century, women are still fighting stereotyping and trying to educate the uninformed about the reality of PMS.

Recently, a lot of publicity has surrounded the male equivalent to PMS, Irritable Male Syndrome (see page 81 for more on IMS): perhaps this discovery will help to discourage the typecasting of women as helpless victims of their hormones – and encourage comediennes to write IMS jokes to liberate us from PMS as man's answer to everything.

*What's the difference between a man with IMS and a jackass? Aftershave.*

Part of the challenge of coping with PMS is to ensure that it doesn't become a way of minimizing us or our feelings. There are hundreds of great coping tools you can learn and lifestyle changes you can make to take control of your life and reduce the impact that PMS has on it.

## Take it Like a Man

Until some brilliant woman designs a PMS simulator, men won't truly understand what millions of us endure each month. It's virtually impossible for a man to imagine a biological syndrome that affects organs he doesn't possess. It's like women trying to empathize with the agony of getting kicked in the family jewels. Nonetheless, if the man in your life is really interested in comprehending his damsel's monthly distress, try explaining it to him this way:

**Your urethra is engorged with blood and tissue, and swollen to the size of a football.** Each and every month this blood and tissue accumulate and make your testicles balloon, your groin cramps, your hands puff to the size of baseball mitts and your desire to go to the office or swing a golf club – or do much of

anything — disappears; you are reduced to a lethargic couch lump (more than usual anyway), who cries when he gets a flat or "snaps" when the Slims Jims® are gone. Even your sex drive is nonexistent. The only thing throbbing is your head.

The payoff to all this "biology" is that you will ultimately hemorrhage through your penis for 3-8 days, stain several tighty whiteys and your favorite gym shorts. Meanwhile, your significant other will be totally insensitive and grumble something like, "You'd think you would've learned to cope with this by now...Let's have sex!"

# If Men Had PMS...

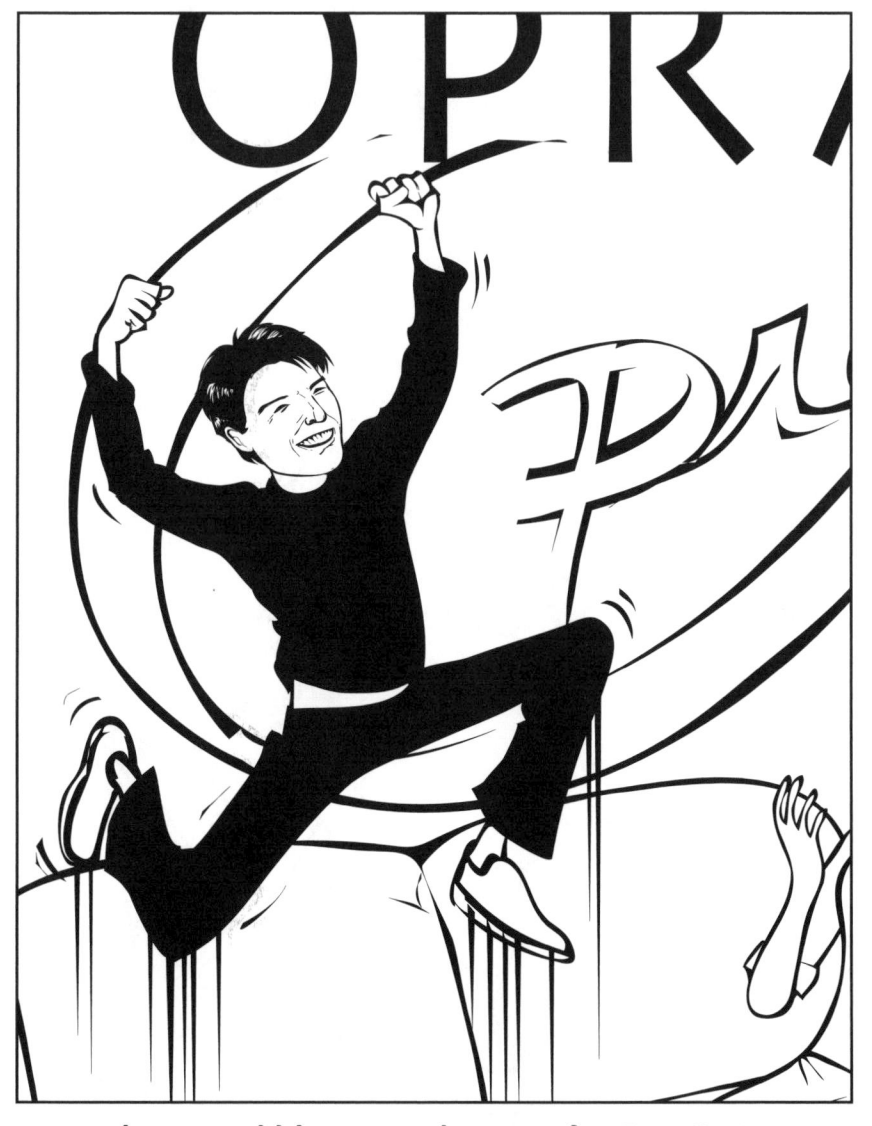

...there would be an explanation for Tom Cruise.

# If Men Had PMS...

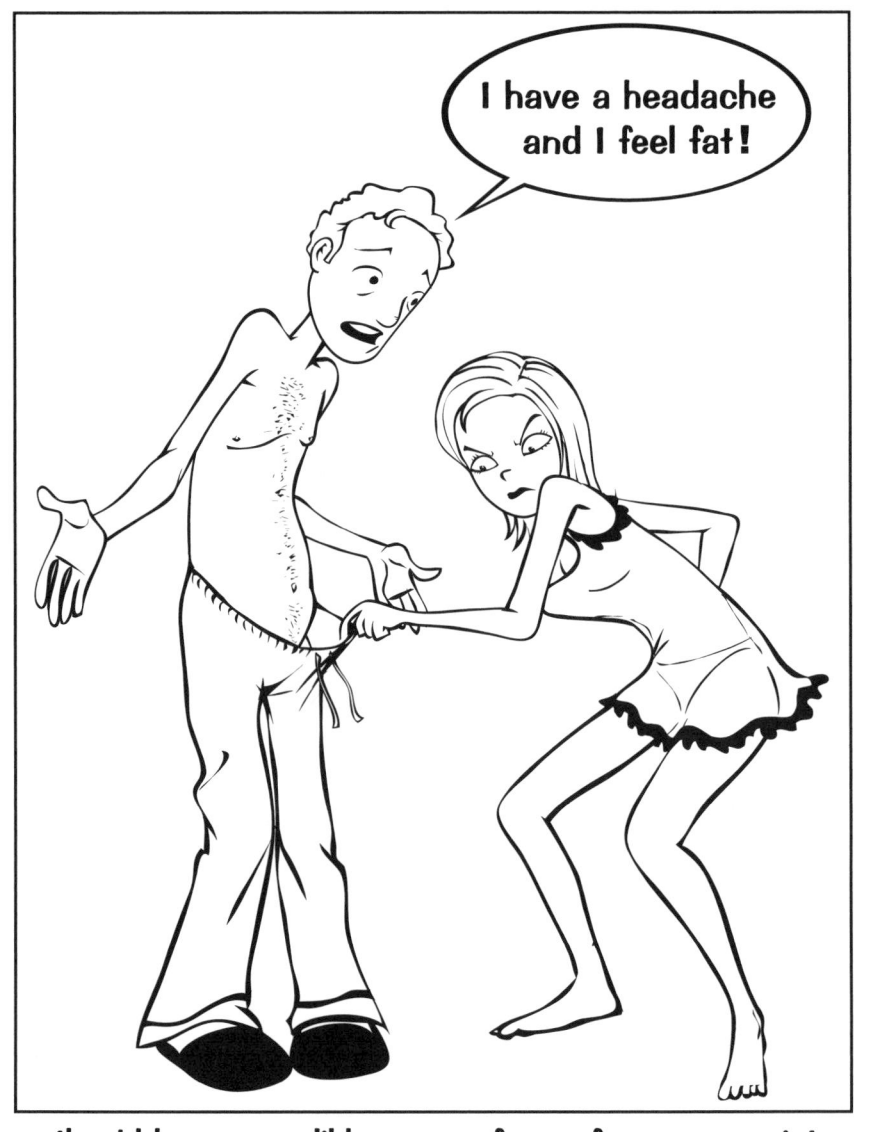

...they'd have a credible excuse for performance anxiety.

# If Men Had PMS...

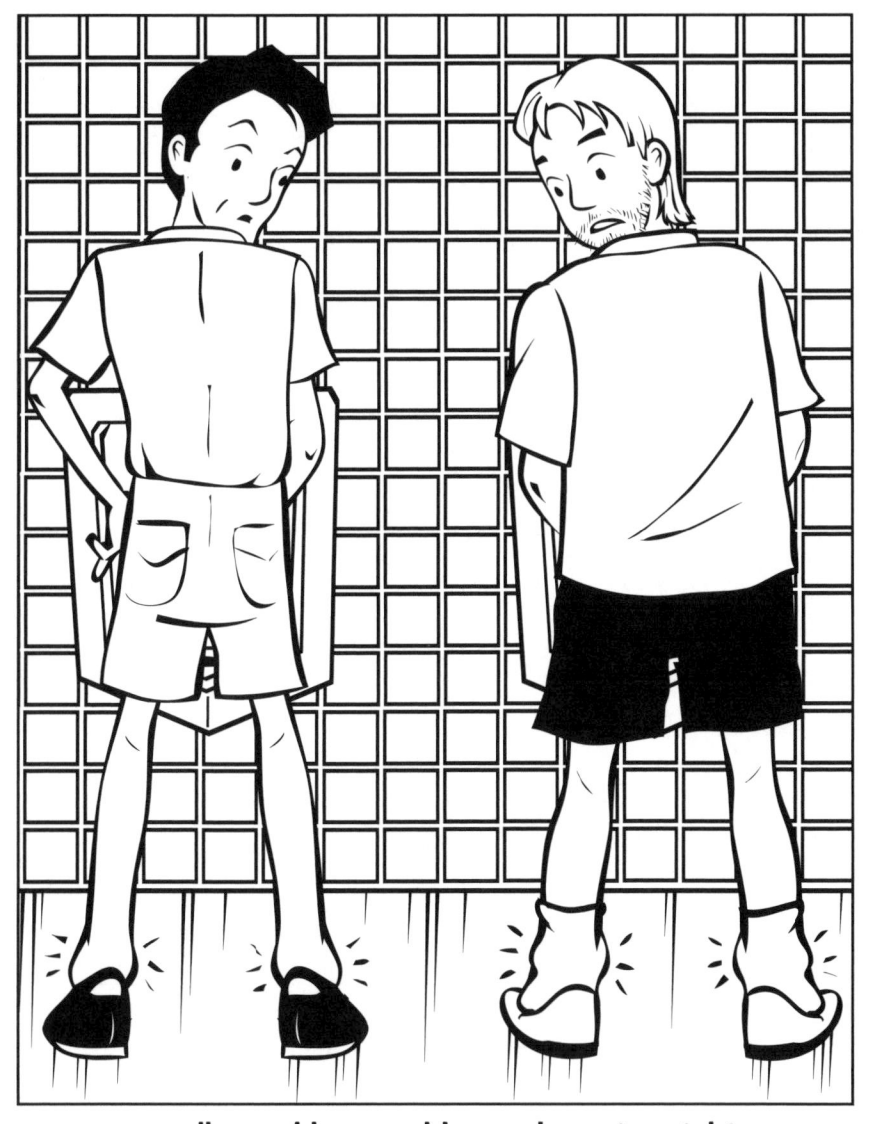

...swollen ankles would earn bragging rights.

*An inexperienced young husband perplexed by his wife's PMS mood swings buys her a mood ring so he can monitor her unpredictable attitude.*

*He soon discovers that when she's in a good mood, it turns green. When she's in a bad mood, it leaves a big f#\*!ing red mark on his forehead.*

*Maybe next time he'll buy her a diamond.*

# Ms. Jekyll and You Better Hide!

## (Recognizing PMS Symptoms)

Is your headache due to **PMS** or because your mother-in-law has moved into the guest room? Are you consuming anything with an expiration date because of your workload or do you imitate the cookie monster only at certain times of the month?

To some of us – and our loved ones – **PMS** is about as subtle as an anvil falling on our heads. For others, the signs are not as discernible, or could be mistaken for common ailments not associated with menstrual misery. Stress at home or in the workplace can cause physical pain, mood swings, and several other symptoms characteristic of **PMS**. So, how do we know when it's **PMS** or an ex-husband's skinny young girlfriend that's getting us down?

27

# Very Aggravating Factors

Females have around 400 menstrual cycles, decades of reminding some male to "zip up" and five years of hot flashes to look forward to in their lives. Hormonal changes in the body flip the PMS switch to "on." For some of us, PMS begins with menarche (the first menstrual period) while others are spared until their 40s. Below are some of the common PMS triggers:

* Perimenopause (the transition to menopause)
* Discontinuing or changing birth control pills
* Childbirth or termination of a pregnancy
* Toxemia during pregnancy (also called pre-eclampsia; a sharp rise in blood pressure and high protein levels in the urine in the third trimester)
* Tubal ligation ("tying the tubes" or sterilization)
* Trauma
* Seasonal Affective Disorder (the response to decreased light in winter)
* Substantial weight gain or loss
* Amenorrhea (not menstruating)
* Change in diet
* Vitamin B, C and/or E, selenium or magnesium deficiencies

There is evidence to suggest that some women are predisposed to PMS, like thunder thighs or heart-shaped ankle tattoos. A family member with PMS, a family history of alcoholism, women with high estrogen levels or low progesterone levels, and women who are inactive have a higher likelihood of having PMS.

Whatever the cause, the symptoms – like the effects of gravity – frequently become more severe as we get older. Perimenopause, the time before full-fledged menopause when the body slows its reproductive function, can be a particularly tough time for

women with **PMS**. Due to the irregular nature of the menstrual cycle in perimenopause, your **PMS** symptoms may not follow an easily identifiable pattern. The body produces less progesterone and estrogen and ovulates less frequently. (Rev up those electric razors, girls!)

# Crash Course: Perimenopause 101

John A. Sunyecz, M.D., F.A.C.O.G.
Specialist in women's reproductive health and menopause

Having PMS makes you more likely to suffer the ravages of perimenopausal symptoms. Perimenopause, the transitional phase before menstruation stops, is marked by changes in the menstrual cycle along with other physical and emotional symptoms, similar to those experienced with PMS (see the list of PMS symptoms on page 34). Perimenopause occurs as the ovaries' production of hormones fluctuates and declines. While it can be a confusing and difficult time for women, it is a natural part of aging that signals the end of their reproductive years.

The average age of menopause in the United States is 51 to 52 years of age, but perimenopause may start as early as 40 to 45 years of age and last from two to eight years. In general, the later in life your perimenopause symptoms begin, the shorter the transition to menopause. During this time, you may experience a combination of PMS and menopausal symptoms or no symptoms at all. However, if you're one of the women who has significant premenstrual symptoms at 30 to 40 years of age, you are more likely to have perimenopausal symptoms.

## Signs and Symptoms

In the early stages of perimenopause, you may see a break in regular cycling of your period; later perimenopause is classified as missing three to 11 months of your period, while menopause is reached after 12 months of no menstrual flow. Shorter cycles and heavier flow are typical indicators of perimenopause. However, it's important to note that a change in your cycle may not mean that you are going through perimenopause; instead, it could be caused by diet, lifestyle, weight loss or gain, exercise level or stress.

The peaks and valleys of estrogen production during perimenopause can cause significant hot flashes and night sweats. These hot flashes may be the classic, intense ones that leave women drenched afterwards, or they may be milder with a sensation of warmth and minor sleep disturbances.

Emotional changes are as common in perimenopause as during PMS and may include irritability, anxiety, depression, fatigue, and frustration. While hormonal fluctuations cause these symptoms, balancing a career, marriage, children and/or other relationships, responsibilities and the stressors of daily life certainly play a role.

## Treatment

With so many common symptoms, such as irritability, joint aches and fatigue, it's not surprising that many of the treatments for PMS work for perimenopause, too. Like PMS, however, there is no magic bullet or single treatment that works well for everyone. The best solution is to treat your most troublesome symptoms.

Depending upon your health history, your healthcare provider may recommend oral contraceptives, which can minimize

fluctuations in estrogen levels. Studies have shown that low-dose birth control pills can provide relief of perimenopausal symptoms, such as hot flashes, mood changes and night sweats. They also regulate the menstrual cycle, provide effective contraception, protect against ovarian and endometrial cancers and prevent bone loss. Many physicians recommend "bicycling" the pill during perimenopause: Women take 42 active pills followed by 7 placebo (sugar) pills. This reduces the number of periods by half and provides very effective perimenopause symptom control.

Years of clinical research have also shown that supplements such as Black Cohosh reduce hot flashes, night sweats and related sleeplessness, irritability and mood swings. Red Clover is also effective for hot flashes and night sweats, and Valerian Root can help with insomnia. For more about these supplements and others, many of which work for the symptoms of PMS and perimenopause, see "It's a Balancing Act: PMS & Supplements" on page 65.

# PMS, the Poser

Recognizing the fire-breathing, Post-It® pasting (try it...it's very satisfying to vent on those little yellow squares and slap them down in strategic places!) two-headed ogre called PMS takes a bit of humble self-reflection. Since PMS comes disguised in many mildly upsetting to horrifying masks and presents in limitless combinations, "werewolf" may seem a likely explanation before "premenstrual syndrome" occurs to you.

Think about it. The large number of symptoms, all of which can occur as part of other illnesses, can even happen to men. After all, guys get backaches and, though they'd have us believe

otherwise, they get irritable and moody, too. So, that nagging headache of yours could be related to stress, diet, allergies, depression, chemical sensitivity, vitamin deficiency or your "Abandon Ship" ranking on Cosmo's "When Mr. Right is All Wrong" quiz. What characterizes it as PMS is *its monthly reoccurrence before menstruation*. Remember, symptoms related to PMS will occur only in the second half of your menstrual cycle and disappear before your period ends. In other words, if you're snorting powdered sugar all month long, you have issues other than PMS.

Although lab work can reliably establish hormone levels, there is no diagnostic test for PMS other than the petrified or pitying looks you get from those around you. In truth, we're better able to assess our changes in health and mood than our healthcare practitioners, who we see infrequently. Before managing your PMS, you'll have to establish the patterns of symptoms you experience and when they occur.

To effectively track your PMS, you'll need to be aware of and monitor your lifestyle, feelings, urges and behavior, and burn the evidence later. You may find that some symptoms you've pegged as PMS-related also occur at other times of the month. Or, you may discover that you're adding chocolate chips to your chicken salad only premenstrually. Once you have a record of your symptoms over two or more menstrual cycles, you'll be armed with all the information you need to gain control of them. We've included a sample PMS tracking chart (the "Monthly 'Monstrual' Chart") and six months of blank ones for you to use on page 137.

# PMDD: No Laughing Matter

A small number of women, perhaps five percent, have Premenstrual Dysphoric Disorder ("PMDD"), classified as a depressive disorder since 1993. By separating PMDD from PMS, medical and mental health professionals are acknowledging that some women have very severe, potentially disabling and sometimes life-threatening symptoms that need appropriate treatment.

While the emotional symptoms of PMS are serious and unpleasant, PMDD may include social withdrawal, inability to work, and even suicidal thoughts, and does require proper intervention. Anti-depressant and anti-anxiety medications have proven to be the most effective treatments. If you suspect you have PMDD, please consult your doctor or mental health practitioner right away.

# Be A PMS Detective

So, besides the water-retentive, pimply obvious, what should you look for? While you are unlikely to experience only one of the 150 or so documented symptoms, you would be a medical miracle – and one miserable PMS mess – if you had them all. Most of us have a combination of physical, behavioral and emotional changes. Following is a partial list of premenstrual symptoms, some of which may sound all too familiar:

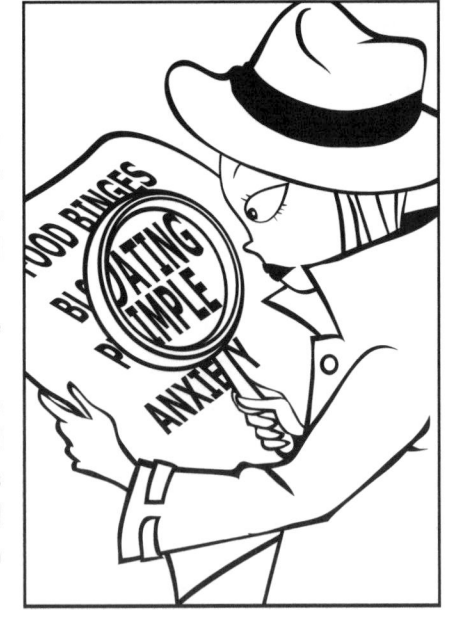

abdominal bloating or cramping
absentmindedness
accident-proneness
acne
alcohol sensitivity
allergies
anger
anxiety
backaches
breast swelling
breast tenderness or pain
confusion
cravings for sweets or salt
crying
depression
dizziness
eating disorders
edema (swelling)
fainting
fatigue
food binges
forgetfulness
frequent urination
headaches
hemorrhoid flare-ups
hives
increased appetite

indecisiveness
infections
insomnia
irregular heartbeat
irritability
joint swelling or aches
lack of coordination
lethargy
migraines
mood swings
muscle aches
nausea
noise sensitivity
palpitations
panic
paranoia
rashes
social withdrawal
self-esteem problems
sex drive changes
smell sensitivity
stiff neck
tension
touch sensitivity
violence
water retention
weight gain

Are we having fun yet? Some premenstrual problems may influence the presence or severity of others. For example, if you typically have eating binges, you're also likely to suffer from weight gain and loss of self-esteem. If you tend toward premenstrual depression, you may also experience social withdrawal, lethargy and a change in sex drive. Symptoms can be interrelated, and that's part of deciphering the complexity of **PMS**.

# Root Canal Is Fun - PMS Sucks!

No two women experience their "first time" or PMS in exactly the same way. You may have friends who share the same symptoms but our life experiences and physiology influence how we react to them. Still, there are millions of women out there who are just as pissed off, achy and tired as you are.

Here, you'll find some of the most common complaints of the PMS hit parade and hear from women who are affected.

## ABDOMINAL CRAMPING

*66 For five or six days before my period even starts, I have horrible cramps. They start with a pulling feeling in my pelvic region, but before long, they've spread to my back and upper thighs. When I was young, I thought women only got cramps during their periods. 99*

Premenstrual cramps feel much like menstrual cramps and can begin as early as two weeks before your period (which leaves about six good days a month if you add the week of complaining before their arrival). You may have premenstrual cramps and no menstrual cramps whatsoever, or your cramps might continue until your period ends. They can affect the abdomen, back, vagina, thighs – and anyone within earshot.

## ACNE

*66 Around age 30, I started breaking out before my period. I thought all that was behind me. Now, I'm in my 40s and I share acne treatments with my teenage daughter. About two weeks before my period, I get pimples on my chest, back and chin. My skin seems to change during this time of the month, and even my makeup looks different. 99*

When we think of the good old days of our youth, acne is ranked alongside orthodontic headgear on our nostalgia meters. Although it's one of the most commonly reported **PMS** symptoms, acne is not caused by **PMS**. Women who can play connect the dots with their pimples, however, may find that their skin problems worsen in the premenstrual phase. Women whose skin is usually clear may have breakouts, and some report that they develop allergies to makeup in the days before their periods. The bright side: If zits form the shape of Mother Teresa, or any of the 12 apostles, you could end up on Montel.

## ANGER, ANXIETY, CRYING, DEPRESSION, IRRITABILITY, LOW SELF-ESTEEM, VIOLENCE (a.ka. Lions and tigers and bears, oh my!)

“*Everything sets me off: TV commercials, people trying to be helpful, people being unhelpful. I dread this time of the month and feel like a zombie. I cry all the time, can't focus on my work, and have more mood swings than I can count. The rest of the month, I'm a happy person. What's wrong with me?*”

If, after ordering enough fast food to feed a Boy Scout troop, you've made the teenage manager cry because your Diet Coke® was flat, you may be a smidgen irritable. It is the emotional symptoms of PMS that most often cause women to seek help outside their refrigerators. The toll on friends, work, family, pets and paper boys can be overwhelming.

The likely source of the turmoil is an imbalance of estrogen and progesterone (remember the vanilla and chocolate of hormones?). An excess of estrogen (vanilla) may cause anxiety (because you need chocolate, too!); an excess of progesterone (chocolate) can cause depression (because it's not a sundae without vanilla). The result: A broken heel can cause a crying jag; an innocent

remark may result in a 10-minute tirade; and, an empty carton of ice cream could set off a chain reaction too horrible to imagine!

**66** *I feel like at any moment I could lose control. I resent taking care of my family for two weeks a month when the truth is that I love them dearly. I spend the other two weeks trying to make up for everything I've done – or haven't done – during PMS.* **99**

These are not the words of a serial killer, but a teacher and mother of three. Women who are nurturing mothers may fear losing control around their children. Women in healthy relationships may feel inexplicable hatred towards their partners. (Note: This last symptom may have nothing to do with PMS!) Family and friends suspect that they can't do anything right, or anything to help – or no longer want to try. If you experience any of these symptoms premenstrually, you may also feel guilty for your behavior or feelings after the symptoms disappear with the onset of your period. We'll talk more about handling these feelings and how they affect our relationships in "Love Me Tender...and Bloated" on page 77.

## BREAST SWELLING, TENDERNESS OR PAIN

**66** *At night, I can't bear the sheets touching my breasts, which become swollen and lumpy. Even my underarms are tender. I feel shooting pains for about a week before my period starts.* **99**

Your significant other may think that breast swelling is the only PMS pro, but it's not sexy to us gals. It hurts! Swelling and tenderness can result in extreme sensitivity to the extent that some women cannot wear bras or tight clothing. Breast tissue can become more fibrous or lumpy, breast cysts (normal and benign) may become enlarged, and some women experience a sensation of heaviness and pain down their arms.

## CRAVINGS FOR SWEET OR SALTY FOOD – OR BOTH!

*" The night before my son's birthday, I ate his cake. I had to get up early the next morning to buy a new one. Who does this? It's like I'm possessed. There isn't enough sugar in the world to satisfy my cravings when I have PMS. Then, I pay for it the rest of the month trying to lose all the weight I've gained. "*

Hormonal changes during the premenstrual phase can result in strong food cravings, just as in pregnancy. Women with pre-existing eating disorders, such as bulimia, often find that the cycle of bingeing and purging increases premenstrually. These days, many of us are on diets and PMS food urges can be disruptive and discouraging. Unfortunately, potato chips as a vegetable substitute are never going to fly!

## FATIGUE

*" Getting out of bed is almost more than I can bear. I try to schedule work or social activities around my exhaustion because I know I'm useless for those days. I'm doing my best, but I'm afraid I'll lose my job."*

For some women with PMS, fatigue can be debilitating. They call in sick to work, send the kids to school half-dressed, and spend the days leading up to their periods napping, or wishing they were. This is not a sign of a secret double life and can occur without depression or any other mood disturbances.

## HEADACHES

*" I wake up with a headache and I go to bed with one. For two weeks a month, I pop pills like candy. My doctor offered to check my eyes or test for food allergies. What's the point? The rest of the month, I'm fine."*

Many women find that tension headaches or migraines occur with greater frequency not only when listening to "on-hold" music, but also in the premenstrual phase of their cycle. Others note that headaches begin with the onset of their periods and last one or two days. If your headaches begin with your period, they're still related to your hormones, but are not **PMS**. If they come on regularly during foreplay, refer to the cure for "hysteria" on page 17.

## SEX DRIVE CHANGES

**" *I love my boyfriend. We have a great relationship, but for two weeks every month, I sleep on the couch. Not only do I not want to have sex, I don't want him near me. He's very understanding, but I know he's frustrated. He's not alone.* "**

Some women experience hypersexuality in the days before their periods, masturbate frequently and feel out of control. Interestingly, their mates don't perceive these symptoms as problems. Others, who have enjoyable sex lives the rest of the month, cannot stand any kind of intimacy. Changing levels of estrogen and testosterone are the culprits.

## WATER RETENTION

**" *I'm a walking reservoir. I swear, sometimes I think people can hear a splashing noise when I'm near. My tummy feels like a water balloon, and my ankles disappear entirely. Stick a pin in me!* "**

If your fingers resemble sausages or strangers keep asking you when you're due – and you're not – water retention may be a problem. Some **PMS** sufferers retain so much water premenstrually, they have two sets of clothes. Water may collect in the ankles, hands, face or abdomen. Water retention and associated weight gain may cause mood swings, self-esteem issues and even depression. Usually, the first day of your period brings significant relief.

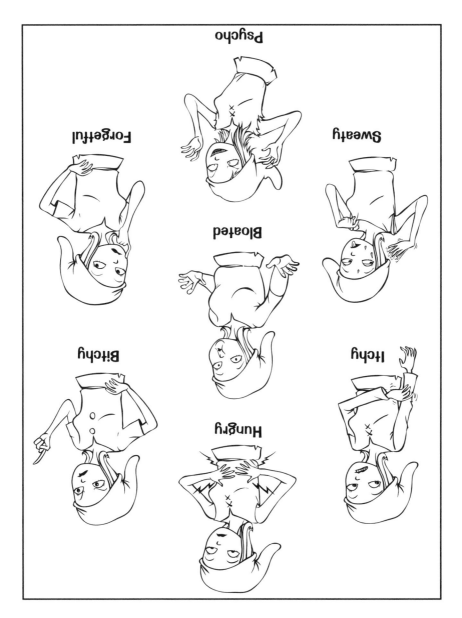

The Princess and the PMS

The Seven PMS Dwarves...

# Don't Stress It

Many studies have suggested that stress can increase the severity of PMS. Negative life changes, such as divorce, job loss, a move or outgrowing your "skinny jeans," may affect your symptoms and how you experience them.

The similarities between PMS symptoms and the body's stress response have prompted further investigation by researchers. Under stress, adrenal glands crank out hormones like cortisol, which can upset the delicate balance of other hormones in the body causing headaches, panic attacks, fatigue, skin problems and digestive upset. Adding insult to injury, high levels of stress hormones can aggravate existing premenstrual symptoms or lead to PMM (see "Another Set of Ominous Initials" below).

You can help yourself and your PMS by dealing with the stressful issues in your life. By becoming more attuned to how you respond to stress, you'll also be more aware of the changes you experience during your menstrual cycle. Developing new coping skills, practicing relaxation techniques and improving your overall health through diet and exercise will prevent stress from turning you into the poster girl for PMS. Learn how to relax and put your PMS-self first in "PMS: A License to Chill" on page 101.

# Another Set of Ominous Initials

Researchers finally realized that the hormonal fluctuations during the luteal (a.k.a. "Get out of the house!") phase of the menstrual cycle have a trickle-down effect. They call it Premenstrual Magnification ("PMM") because it increases the severity or frequency of underlying health issues, such as asthma, epilepsy, herpes, digestive problems, infections, eating disorders and other serious

ailments, for a double dose of discomfort. Unfortunately, some healthcare practitioners have trouble grasping the concept and women who complain of worsening symptoms before their periods are often met with the same head-scratching that PMS sufferers endured 40 years ago.

The only way to tell if you suffer from PMM is to track your symptoms, noting when they occur, how severe they are and how long they last. Both PMS and PMM can be present at the same time. To avoid confusion when tracking your symptoms, remember that PMS symptoms occur only premenstrually and disappear with the onset of your period. PMM symptoms worsen premenstrually but improve slowly with the onset of your period. They don't disappear entirely.

If, for example, you have infrequent asthma attacks until days before your period, and tracking shows that, month after month, the frequency and/or severity increases as your period approaches, this information should be shared with your physician. He or she may be able to adjust the timing or dosage of medication to help control the underlying condition.

## When it's Not PMS

Meet mittelschmerz. No, it's not a relative of Beetlejuice or a new gourmet cheese. Mittelschmerz (pronounced MITT-ul-shmurz) is the pain associated with ovulation and clinicians say that about 20% of women experience it. There are several explanations for the German word that literally means "middle pain." At the time of ovulation, fluid or blood is released from the ruptured egg follicle and can cause irritation of the abdominal lining.

Mittelschmerz, sneaky devil that it is, may be felt on one side one month, and then switch to the opposite side the next month. The pain is not harmful and does not signify the presence of disease. It's also not PMS, nor is it a symptom of PMS. If you've consistently been charting your menstrual cycle, as well as your symptoms, it will likely fall outside the range of the hormonal hiccups that are causing your premenstrual pain.

Another source of misery not related to PMS is endometriosis, a condition in which the tissue that lines the uterus, called the endometrium, grows outside of the uterus. It can cause disabling cramps, pelvic and lower back pain, discomfort during sex, intestinal pain and heavy periods. Talk to your doctor if you have any or all of these symptoms.

# Sick or Treat? M.D.s Can Help

As erratic hormone levels leave some of us wondering if we'll suddenly be sprouting chest hairs or hosting a Brownie Troop meeting at Chippendale's®, doctors still search for a cure. They may not have figured out PMS yet, but physicians do have some tools to treat the symptoms. Don't forget to take your "Monthly 'Monstrual' Chart" when you see your doctor. The more information you can provide, the better your physician can treat you.

Following are some treatments your physician may recommend:

✳ Diuretics, or "water pills," help the body eliminate excess fluid through the kidneys. Your doctor may prescribe a diuretic to reduce bloating if restricting your salt intake does not help. Although studies on the benefits of diuretics for PMS have shown mixed results, they have been used in PMS treatment longer than any other medication.

✴ NSAIDs, or Non-Steroidal Anti-Inflammatory medications such as Ponstel®, are sometimes used to relieve premenstrual pain. A variety of over-the-counter NSAIDs are also available, including ibuprofen (Advil®, Motrin IB®) and naproxen (Aleve®). However, all carry a risk of stomach inflammation with ongoing use.

✴ Finally, there are prescription anti-depressants to treat the mood symptoms of PMS. SSRI (Selective Serotonin Reuptake Inhibitor) anti-depressants, such as Zoloft® and Prozac®, increase the amount of serotonin in the brain, which can help to improve moods and alleviate depression. Because SSRIs have a variety of side effects that women already experience with PMS, including insomnia, sexual dysfunction, drowsiness, headache and anxiety, they are best used only by women whose mood symptoms severely impair their ability to function.

✴ There are new products available, such as Yaz®, a birth control pill, that are prescribed to treat the symptoms of PMDD (see more on Premenstrual Dysphoric Disorder on page 33). Be sure to explain all of your symptoms to your physician as well as your PMS treatment plan, including exercise, diet, etc. so that he or she can prescribe the best medication for your needs.

# I Don't Have PMS, I Really Hate You

If, after tracking your symptoms for a few months, you discover that there is no clear premenstrual pattern, you may need to consult a doctor. Whether the root of your problem is physical or psychological, there is no reason for you to continue suffering.

For most women, making the lifestyle modifications suggested in this book will alleviate discomfort. For others, it may take a passport and a European lover, but there's a lot to be said for healthy living.  Then again, if in the course of filling out the "Monthly 'Monstrual' Chart" you learn that you're out of sorts all the time, you might want to make some personal changes and seek the quality of life you deserve.

*"You don't want to cross my path*
*Cause a pitbull ain't no match*
*For these teeth a clenchin', fluid retention*
*Head a swellin', can't stop yellin'*
*Got no patience, I'm so hateful*
*PMS blues, premenstrual syndrome*
*Got those moods a swingin', tears a slingin'*
*Nothin' fits me when it hits me*
*Rantin', ravin', misbehavin' PMS blues"*

*(from "PMS Blues," a song by Dolly Parton)*

# PMS SOS:
# Treating the Symptoms

Once a month, we enter a premenstrual parallel universe where everyday tasks seem monumental and everyone else has a bad attitude. Overnight, the voices of little ones seem extra loud and demanding, a husband's familiar aftershave smells overpowering and vile, and no one can do anything right! Tears flow and emotions careen like a runaway train. And what's more exasperating, it isn't until "the PMS days" pass that we realize – or admit – it was us who derailed.

## For the Pre-Premenstrual...

Prepare the pubescent princess in your house with a PMS Patty Doll... Comes with bloated belly, zit stickers and granny panties. (Hatchet and miniature box of bon-bons sold separately.)

## Fighting the Fetal Position

Whether from pain, depression or fatigue, we would like nothing more than to be left alone until the funk fades. The last thing we want to hear while PMS storm clouds gather overhead is "eat healthy foods and exercise." Well-meaning spouses and friends take their lives in their hands by merely suggesting a walk, let alone a session on a Stairmaster® to "get the blood flowing." However, there is no doubt that what we put into our bodies and the amount of physical activity we do or don't get affect the severity of PMS.

Take heart. We're not prescribing a strict diet, there's no weighing of portions or prepackaged meals to buy and nobody is suggesting you join a thong-thronged gym. On the other hand, this is not a change for the week or two a month that you have PMS. Instead, there are small steps you can take every day that will improve your overall health and your PMS.

The best news is that by following these suggestions, the cravings and fatigue that make it so hard to diet and exercise in the first place will go away. *Yeah, right,* the skeptical among you are thinking. But you'd be surprised what a difference a few adjustments a day make.

# Looking for a Mr. Goodbar (A Sugar Daddy Will Do!)

Comedienne Elaine Boosler once quipped, "We have women in the military, but they don't put us in the front lines. They don't know if we can fight, if we can kill. I think we can. All the general has to do is walk over to the women and say, "You see the enemy over there? They say you look **FAT** in those uniforms! Now kill them." Add PMS to the mix and women would tear the enemy limb from limb.

Of all the four-letter words, "diet" is the one that really makes us cringe. Only the appalling phrases "swimsuit season" and "full price" bring more grown women to their knees. There's so much diet information out there, and the news changes daily. Carbs

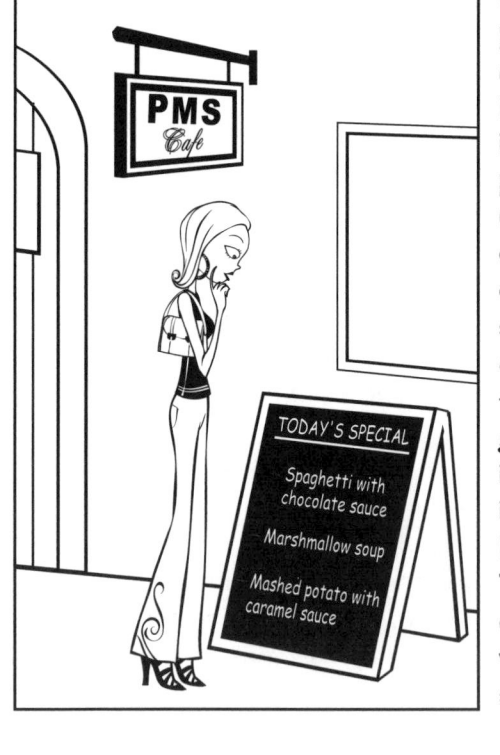

TODAY'S SPECIAL

Spaghetti with chocolate sauce

Marshmallow soup

Mashed potato with caramel sauce

are good, carbs are bad; protein is good, but not too much protein, and so on. But *why* you eat is just as important as *what* you eat, particularly during PMS. Do you answer the siren song of salty chips in the middle of the night or are you a sugar junkie? Are you eating creamy, carb-laden feel-good food for instant gratification, and paying for it later while stuffing yourself into control-top pantyhose? Here's a helping of truth: The food we eat can either drain our energy and aggravate PMS or alleviate the symptoms.

# Healthy Change Isn't a Piece of Cake

Though it may be what we grab for in the depths of PMS, sugar is packed with calories and contains no vitamins, minerals or fiber. Refined sugar causes a spike in your blood sugar then a rapid drop. We've all experienced the sugar crash and burn. A few hours after ingestion, our bodies use up the fuel and the sweet white crystals leave us pawing the pantry for more.

When you miss meals in an effort to lose weight or control cravings, your blood sugar takes a dive and sends you straight for the refined sugars. Almost every study on diet and PMS suggests women eat three meals and three snacks per day. It's hard to believe that the answer is to eat more food, but the question is which food?

# Do it Like the Greeks

Rather than getting a degree in nutrition to make sense of all this, we'd like to introduce you to the Mediterranean Diet – or simply, "what the Greeks eat." The Diet is from the island of Crete where the locals live longer than any other population in the world. They are 20% less likely to die of coronary artery disease and have one-third less cancer than Americans. The Mediterranean Diet is associated with a reduction in joint swelling, aches and pains, which is encouraging for a PMS sufferer from any country. It fits all the criteria for a PMS-friendly eating plan, is tasty and easy to follow.

The idea is to eat more foods from the bottom of the pyramid (on the opposite page) and fewer foods from the top. Grains, vegetables, fruits and protein are more nutritious and because they are digested and metabolized slowly, they give us energy for longer periods of time. These evenly converted fuels make our bodies feel better and run efficiently.

# The Traditional Mediterranean Diet Pyramid

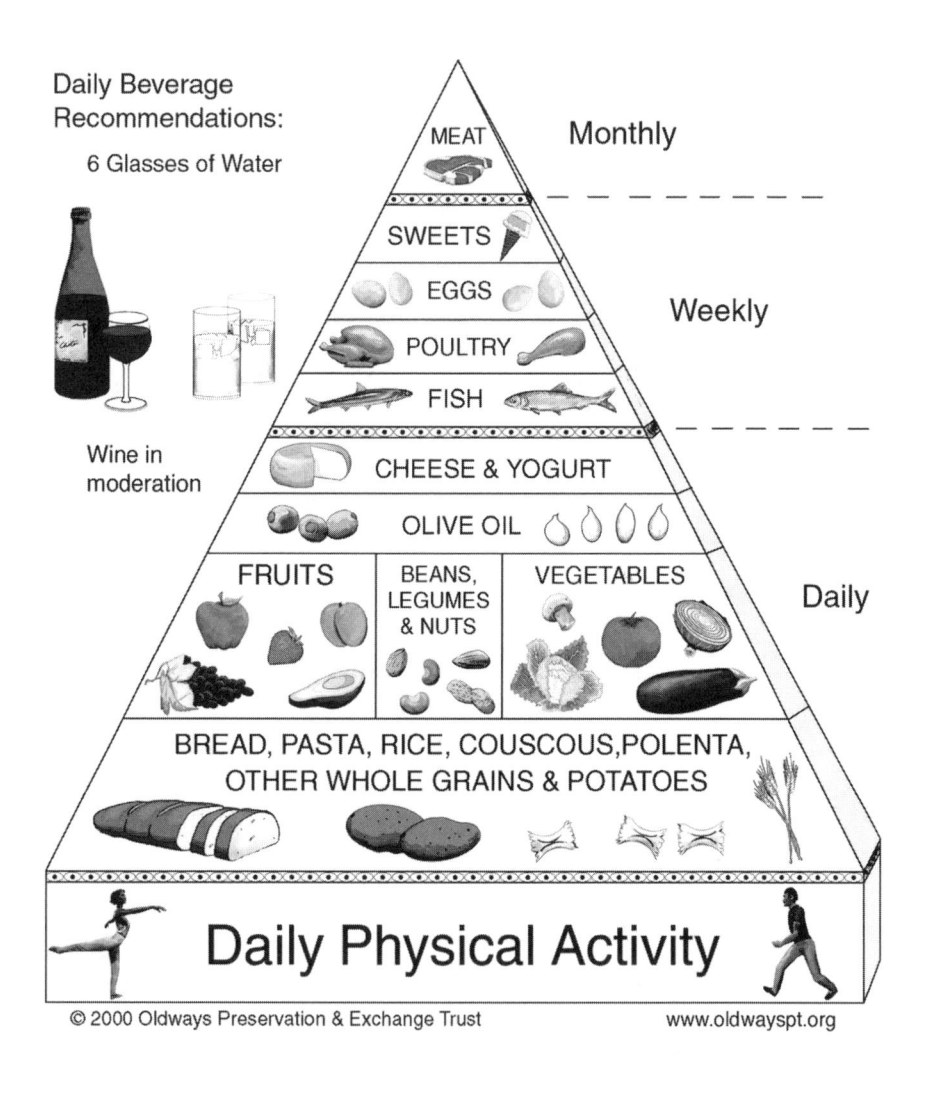

Daily Beverage Recommendations:

6 Glasses of Water

Wine in moderation

MEAT — Monthly

SWEETS
EGGS
POULTRY
FISH — Weekly

CHEESE & YOGURT
OLIVE OIL

FRUITS | BEANS, LEGUMES & NUTS | VEGETABLES — Daily

BREAD, PASTA, RICE, COUSCOUS, POLENTA, OTHER WHOLE GRAINS & POTATOES

Daily Physical Activity

© 2000 Oldways Preservation & Exchange Trust          www.oldwayspt.org

While your current food pyramid may look more like the one below, eating snacks and meals from the Mediterranean Diet pyramid is the quickest route to **PMS** emancipation.

# The Traditional PMS Food Pyramid

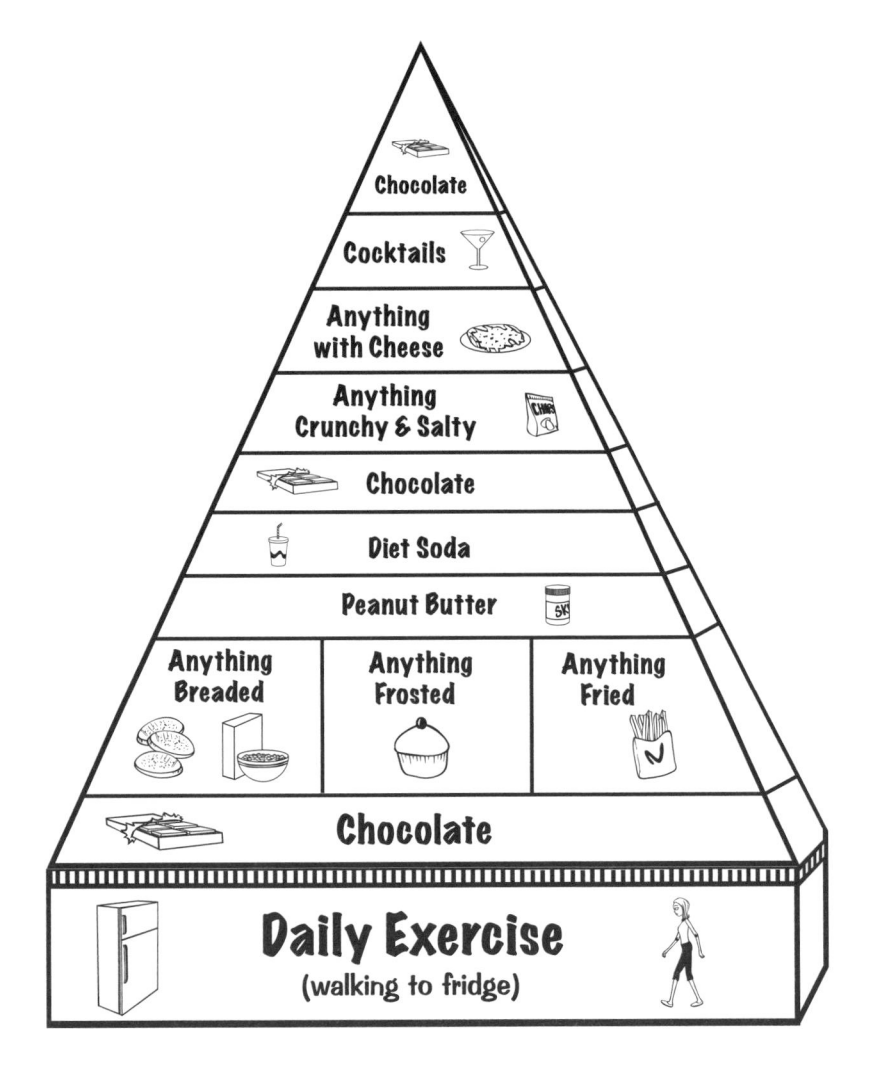

Chocolate

Cocktails

Anything with Cheese

Anything Crunchy & Salty

Chocolate

Diet Soda

Peanut Butter

Anything Breaded

Anything Frosted

Anything Fried

Chocolate

## Daily Exercise
(walking to fridge)

# Let's Make a Meal

The Mediterranean Diet pyramid, like the USDA's version, recommends eating lots of fruits, vegetables and whole grains. However, the Greeks eat far less red meat, and substitute moderate amounts of poultry and cold water fish such as salmon, tuna, mackerel, herring and sardines that contain important omega-3 oils.

The USDA pyramid that we're all familiar with also doesn't distinguish between types of fat: unsaturated, saturated and trans-fat. The Mediterranean Diet contains very little saturated and trans-fat, the building blocks of commercial baked goods, instead focusing on healthier olive oil, olives and nuts. Add low- or non-fat yogurts (without aspartame) feta, ricotta, romano, parmesan and mozzarella cheeses and eat like you're in Crete!

# Fill Her Up!

We know what you're thinking. You've been here before. One too many times you've cleared the kitchen of forbidden food only to find yourself sucking down the expired jar of 3 ½ maraschino cherries – juice and all. Anything to take the edge off the late night transformation that has you jonesing for sweets like a vampire coveting its next victim. But, the fast food freak can be satiated during PMS with some beneficial and tasty foods from the Mediterranean Diet.

Try salads with tomatoes, cucumbers, green peppers, onions, olives and cheese. Throw on roasted or marinated green and red peppers, beets, wild or cultivated greens, cauliflower, cabbage, artichokes, zucchini or eggplant. Dried legumes like

yellow split peas, broad beans, chickpeas and lentils, cooked until tender, can be mashed and mixed with olive oil, onion and salt or can be added into soups. Potatoes are often baked or sautéed in a little olive oil, or steamed with other vegetables for hot or cold combinations. Pasta, barley and rice are seasoned with onions, garlic and spices, and mixed with veggies.

For protein, think grilled fish or poultry brushed with olive oil and garlic; it's quick to prepare and great for the entire family. For dessert, choose seasonal fruit like cherries, honeydew, watermelon, grapes, figs, pomegranates, apples and oranges. At snack time, hit the yogurt with fresh fruit or try a handful of nuts, which will satisfy crunchy cravings, or olives, all of which are surprisingly filling.

Just because it's good for you, doesn't mean it has to taste like cardboard. Changing your eating habits doesn't mean starving, or depriving yourself of all your favorite foods. Small changes over weeks and months are easier to accept and will start you on your recovery from PMS and hopefully, a lifelong habit of healthier eating.

It takes about three months for the change in diet to make a significant impact on PMS symptoms, but you should start feeling the benefits to your overall health and energy level right away. When you feel really good, try reintroducing one or two of the foods you avoided during your recovery phase. Should you start to feel sluggish or achy again, you may choose to say "Adio" ("goodbye" in Greek) to those foods for good. If your PMS is resistant to the Mediterranean Diet, try following the advice of Dr. Neal Barnard on the next page.

# Crash Course: Foods That Work 101

Neal Barnard, M.D.
Specialist and clinical researcher in health & nutrition

A few years ago, a young woman called me to ask for painkillers. Her menstrual cramps were so excruciating that she was unable to do much of anything except lie in bed and wait for her pain to go away. I told her that I would be glad to prescribe painkillers for a few days, but I also suggested that she change her diet, just as an experiment, for the next four weeks. She agreed, and a month later, she called to say that she felt wonderful. The disabling pain that was such a regular feature of her life had not come back.

## The Estrogen Connection

During your monthly cycle, the level of estrogens in your blood rises and falls like a roller coaster. Some foods can smooth out your estrogen shifts and others prevent the amount of estrogen in your blood from climbing too high. When the young woman called to ask for help with menstrual cramps, I simply helped her choose foods that would keep her estrogen level from rising. The goal was to smooth out the hormone roller coaster so that the changes in her uterus wouldn't be so dramatic.

Why not eat the foods that work for you instead of those that work against you? When you avoid animal fat and keep vegetable oils to a minimum, your body makes less estrogen. At the same time, high-fiber foods help your body eliminate excess estrogen more easily. Lower estrogen production is also linked to reduced risk of breast cancer and migraines.

In a study with 19 women at the Department of Obstetrics and Gynecology at Georgetown University School of Medicine, we

asked everyone to avoid all animal products and added oils for two months, and to focus on simple, unprocessed foods, such as rice and other whole grains, beans, vegetables and fruits, making their diet rich in fiber. Most of the women noticed a difference, and for some the change was profound. Their pain was gone or dramatically reduced, something they hadn't experienced for years.

After two months, we asked part of the group to return to their previous diet so we could compare the effects. To our surprise, many were extremely reluctant to do so. They had less pain, more energy and had lost weight. Although it had taken a few weeks to get used to the new way of eating, they had become attached to it. They began to view meat and other fatty foods as the enemies that had caused their problems.

## Putting Food to Work

You can begin making these changes today. The key is to follow the diet exactly, so that you can see the effect it has for you. Like the Mediterranean Diet, you'll be focusing on grains, fruits and vegetables. However, this is a vegan diet, meaning no animal products. For many women, eliminating animal products and other fats can solve the pain and PMS puzzle. If you're willing to give it a try, you should:

**Eat plenty of:**

* Whole grains like brown rice, whole grain bread and oatmeal
* Vegetables, such as broccoli, spinach, carrots, sweet potatoes, Swiss chard, brussels sprout or any others
* Legumes, such as beans, peas and lentils
* Fruits

Avoid completely:

* Animal products of any type, such as fish, poultry, meats, eggs and dairy products
* Added vegetable oils, such as salad dressings, margarine and all cooking oils
* Any other fatty foods, including chips, peanut butter, etc.

This sounds like a significant change, however, most people make it in about two weeks. It is important to avoid animal products and oily foods completely; even modest amounts can cause more symptoms. Those who have the best success experiment with new foods and enlist the support of their friends or partners at home.

As the benefits begin — fewer symptoms, easy weight loss and increased energy — the diet change is so rewarding that you'll wish you'd tried it sooner. Try it for just one menstrual cycle (one month) and you'll see what it can do for you. You'll likely start to look at the power of foods in a very different way.

## Starbucks® Has Decaf, Too

It's been said that the more complicated the order at a gourmet coffee shop ("I'll have a triple espresso with a splash of skim milk, a double squirt of raspberry syrup, 2 ½ Sweet'n Lows® in an extra large cup to go") the bigger the jerk ordering it. So why not improve your health and your social standing by simply saying, "Decaf, please."

Caffeine comes from many different sources: your morning coffee, sodas, energy drinks, tea, chocolate and even medications like Midol®, Aqua-Ban® and Excedrin® — the holy trinity of the PMS arsenal. Caffeine can make you anxious, sleepless, jittery and hyper-alert; it also plays a role in breast tenderness and reduces levels of important minerals like calcium and magnesium.

Researchers have discovered that caffeine blocks the brain chemical adenosine, which causes nerve receptors to become hyperactive. In other words, if you're irritable, you'll feel more irritable and if you're stressed, caffeine will make you more stressed. Add PMS, and it's a recipe for head-spinning disaster.

If you're a soda addict, switching to decaf and sugar-free varieties may not help. Women who consume lots of NutraSweet® and Equal® (aspartame), the sugar-substitute most frequently found in soft drinks, report symptoms including depression, irritability, sugar cravings, headaches and poor sleep patterns. Sound familiar?

If you've switched to decaf but still gorge on all things chocolate, you're not out of the woods. Caffeine in any form sucks magnesium out of you like fat through a lipo-wand. Magnesium regulates muscle relaxation and blood sugar and promotes sound sleep – all critical during PMS. Magnesium also increases calcium absorption in the body. A study in The American Journal of Obstetrics and Gynecology reported that 1,200 mg a day of chewable calcium carbonate reduced symptoms of PMS by nearly 50 percent. Another study found that 200 mg a day of magnesium reduced fluid retention, breast tenderness and bloating by 40 percent.

Weaning yourself off caffeine isn't something you'd want to do twice, so make the transition slowly. Reduce your intake of caffeine by a third every few days. But first, you might want to warn loved ones – with a neon sign or a t-shirt emblazoned with "Approach at your own risk!" Rapid withdrawal from caffeine can cause mind-bending headaches and legendary crankiness. To be safe, begin your caffeine reduction program on the first or second day of your period rather than during PMS. Women report some improvement to their PMS symptoms in the first month without caffeine and dramatic improvement by the third month.

# Dousing the PMS Demons

When we're puffed up like blowfish, the last thing we want is more liquid. But, water actually helps reduce premenstrual joint swelling and bloating. You've heard it before and it's still true: Drink six to eight 8-ounce glasses of water every day. Avoid tap water whenever possible, as it contains contaminants and heavy metals. Bottled or filtered water is best.

Dr. Hyla Cass recommends the following in her book *Eight Weeks to Vibrant Health:* Fill up a 64-ounce bottle with water and refill your cup from it throughout the day until it's gone. Water is much better absorbed and utilized when you sip it throughout the day rather than gulp down a glass or two every few hours. Drink more if you like – this is only the minimum. Just make sure you're within sprinting distance of a restroom. You can substitute non-caffeinated herbal teas, too.

# Munch Break

Many of us develop psychological and even physical dependence on certain foods or drinks, whether it's caffeine to wake us up, comfort food to calm us down, or a Jell-O® shot to work up the nerve for another wet t-shirt contest. So, if you'd contemplate giving up sex before doing without your morning leaded coffee or you spend hours fantasizing about fried mozzarella sticks, you need them a tad more than you should.

Once you are on a nutritious diet, amazingly most cravings will disappear, leaving you free to choose one cookie for dessert, rather than devouring a box of them. Changing habits or a pattern of dependence takes time. Remind yourself that the changes you're choosing to make are difficult but necessary steps toward a long-term goal: Brad Pitt buck-naked on your futon. Okay, probably not going to happen, but would you settle for a break from PMS?

# Curb Your Enthusiasm for Stimulants

Dr. Cass has a quick tip to stop cravings for fast food, sugar, chocolate, alcohol or caffeine. She advises keeping a bottle of capsules of the amino acid L-glutamine on hand (check your local health food store or www.pmscentral.com). When a craving strikes, try pouring the contents directly under your tongue to send your food urges packing. L-Glutamine is absorbed quickly and can give you an almost instant pick-me-up similar to your longed-for stimulant. Many women take L-glutamine several times a day, between meals, to prevent cravings. As with all supplements, it's best to check with your own doctor first.

# Move (and Improve!) Your Groove Thing

Besides putting on makeup and/or a bra, exercise is probably the last thing you feel like doing when the cramps set up camp. Even so, several studies have proven the benefit of regular, moderate exercise for women with PMS. The best time to start is now, but if you feel that snow in July is more likely than you getting motivated in the midst of a bad PMS bout, then start after your next period.

Exercise will help you to maintain or lose weight, minimize bloating, reduce cramps and improve self-esteem. It can also do wonders for your stress level. In fact, many women find that once they establish an exercise routine, they feel irritable or unsettled on the days they don't work out. You'll only believe the previous sentence when you experience it for yourself; otherwise all you'll read is "blah, blah, blah, blah!" But it's true because when we exercise, endorphins, the same chemical our brains release during sex, produce a natural high that relieves premenstrual discomfort.

Start simply if exercise is a foreign concept. Take a walk, a beginner's aerobics class or go for a swim. Try to incorporate things you like: if you're a nature girl, exercise outdoors; if you love music, learn to salsa or two-step. It matters less what you do and more that you enjoy it. Exercise is like sex, the more pleasure you take from it, the more likely it is that you'll continue doing it. If you're a social butterfly, ask some friends to join you. For individual challenges, think about running, horseback riding or biking.

If you've been sedentary for a while, begin with 20 minutes each day. To get the greatest benefit from exercise, you need at least 30 minutes per day of vigorous exercise, four days a week. That means you need to break a sweat, and quitting Snickers® bars cold turkey doesn't count. Ultimately, you should do as much exercise as you can, without overdoing it. As you build muscle, you'll find that your metabolism increases and your body burns more fat. You'll be a lean, mean, PMS-free machine who feels a whole lot better about herself and her derriere.

## File NEPA Under "Duh"

NEPA stands for Non-Exercise Physical Activity and is just a nifty way of saying "move." NEPA is the key to lifelong fitness. It means taking the stairs instead of the elevator, parking further away from your destination, doing squats while you're watching TV, stretching while you're standing in line at the bank or waiting for the oven timer to ring. Even gardening, walking the dog and vacuuming count toward a PMS-liberated you. So does sex, but that may not be on the menu until some of your other symptoms have been resolved. Incorporating exercise into your daily activities is easy. Women are the best multi-taskers, after all.

## Step Up to the Mat

Yoga is an ancient discipline that involves stretching, flexibility, strength-building movement, breathing exercises and various types of relaxation techniques. It's also a great way to bring a little PMS peace into your life. In the past 10 years, yoga has gone from an exotic practice to a national health craze, with dozens of types being taught all across the U.S.

If you're looking for a low-impact, rhythmic type of yoga, choose Hatha, gentle yoga or flow yoga. If you want a physically challenging workout, consider power or Ashtanga yoga, Iyengar or Bikram®. Most yoga studios will let you take one or two trial classes before signing up, so try a few to see which one is right for you. Or, try one of the many excellent videos and practice in the privacy of your own home if you – or your sweats – are not quite fit for public viewing during PMS.

## Bark Back at the Beast

It's time to cancel your subscription to Soldier of Fortune Magazine® and enjoy life all month long. We know that PMS can be a debilitating, miserable experience but it won't get any better if you don't make some adjustments. That's why you're reading this book, because you believe in the possibility of change.

Use the tracking charts at the back of the book to follow your own progress. We promise that you'll feel better, have more energy and see a reduction in your PMS symptoms within a few months. Given a chance, our bodies will choose health over sickness. Aren't you curious to see if these changes will help? After all, you've got nothing to lose but your symptoms!

# PMS Day Planner

Here's an example of a day that promotes premenstrual health:

* 6:30 a.m. – Begin your day with some deep breaths and stretching exercises to get your blood flowing.

* 7:00 a.m. – Make time for a breakfast of whole grain bread or cereal, skim milk, some fruit and herbal tea. Pack your lunch and snacks for the day.

* 10:00 a.m. – Mid-morning snack of low-fat yogurt, fruit or a handful of almonds. Don't forget to sip from your water bottle to keep hydrated.

* 11:30 a.m. – Stressed? Take 10 deep, slow breaths.

* 12:30 pm – Nutritious lunch of a salad with some chicken or fish, lots of fresh veggies and a little cheese. Take a 15-minute walk with a friend or coworker to decompress.

* 2:00 p.m. & 4:00 p.m. – More fruit or nut snacks to keep your blood sugar up.

* 6:00 p.m. – Keep dinner healthy and simple, and ask family members to help out with a little clean up.

* 7:45 p.m. – Take 30 to 45 minutes for yourself and do whatever relaxes you. Try a bath, listen to music, go for a walk or write in your journal.

* 8:45 p.m. – A light snack keeps blood sugar from dropping overnight.

* 9:30 p.m. – Take a few minutes to prepare and prioritize your goals for the next day.

* 10:00 p.m. – Getting to bed early when you're premenstrual helps you battle fatigue.

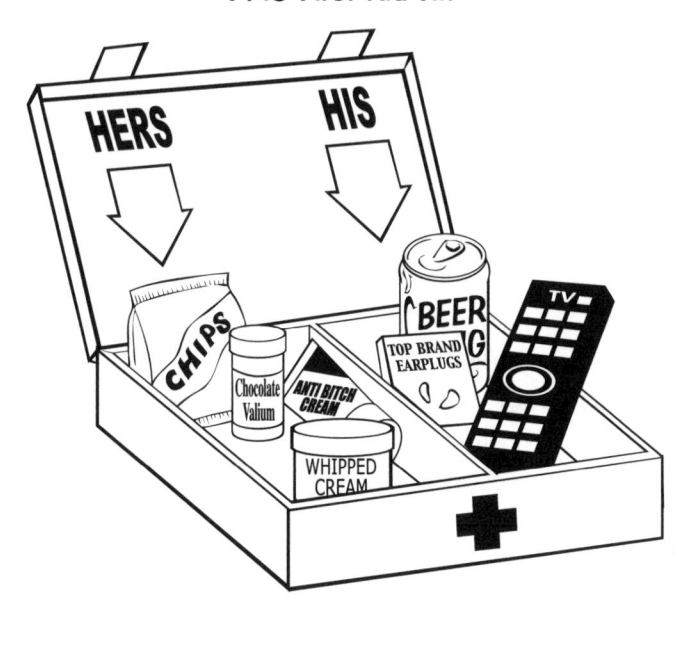

# It's a Balancing Act: PMS & Supplements

Legendary rocker Mick Jagger had the right idea when he sang about hard-working women who needed a little "assistance" with their daily routines: "...She goes running for the shelter of a mother's little helper/And it helps her on her way, gets her through her busy day..." Although he wasn't exactly referring to a vitamin boost for harried moms in the mid-1960s, in the 21st century that's most likely what women need – especially when PMS hits home.

Women may be tough, but we're also frequently vitamin deficient. A steady diet of "seefood" (whatever you see, you eat) can cause some alarming gaps in nutrition, but as you make discerning food choices, many of your vitamin and mineral deficiencies will be corrected. However, there are supplements that you can take to provide additional relief for your more menacing symptoms.

# Not a Bitter Pill

Vitamins, minerals, amino acids and plant-based (herbal) remedies have all shown great promise in the treatment of **PMS**. They are generally kinder to the body than modern pharmaceuticals and remain a primary treatment for illness in many cultures.

Nonetheless, a trip to your local health food store can leave you overwhelmed and confused with the literally thousands of supplements for everything from brittle nails to broken hearts. Many have strange names and stranger ingredients. Don't be fooled into thinking that they're all good for you, or even necessary. The supplement industry is driven by profits and largely unregulated by the FDA. So, a dose of caution with your daily vitamins is highly recommended.

You will usually see the benefits of supplements by the third menstrual cycle (if not sooner) while many of the herbs provide more immediate relief. However, natural doesn't always mean safe, particularly if you're taking prescription medication. On page 148, we've included a quick reference chart of remedies and precautions, but it's always safest to check with your doctor. If you experience an adverse reaction, contact your healthcare provider immediately.

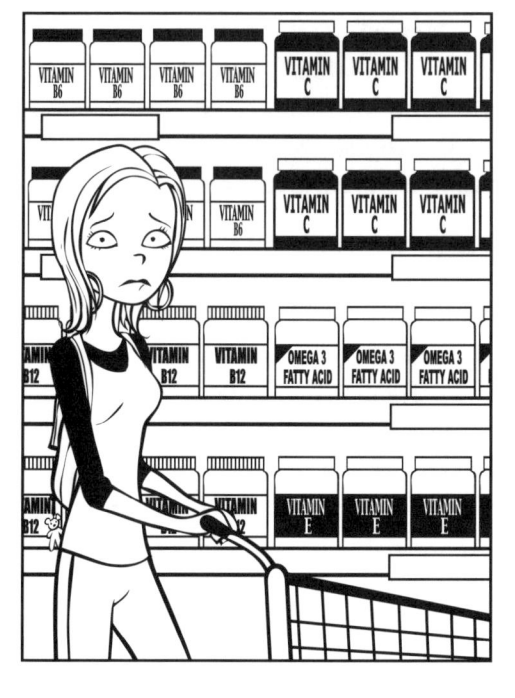

# Vitamins & Minerals

Look for a balanced multi-vitamin formulated for PMS relief, but be aware most multivitamins will not have enough calcium to help with your PMS. For best results, take your vitamins all month long, not only during PMS. While all vitamins and minerals are important for your health, the ones that follow are especially helpful in treating your premenstrual symptoms.

## CALCIUM

We've all heard about the bone-building benefits of calcium, but it's also a calming agent that can be depleted by stress. Several scientific studies have shown that women treated with calcium experienced a 50% reduction in their PMS symptoms, including pain, depression and food cravings. Doctors caution that your body can't absorb more than 500 mg at a time, so keep that in mind, and try taking a dose with each meal. Calcium can also be found in fortified orange juice and all dairy products.

## MAGNESIUM

Like calcium, magnesium calms the nervous system and can relieve muscle spasms, anxiety, constipation and water retention.

However, too much can act as a laxative so it's best taken in divided doses wtih meals. Look for the chelated forms of magnesium, which are more easily absorbed. Beet greens, lima beans, black beans, Swiss chard, tofu, pineapple, raspberries, almonds, sunflower seeds and whole grains are great sources of magnesium in your diet.

## VITAMIN B6

Vitamin B6 helps keep the central nervous system working smoothly. Studies have shown that B6 can relieve bloating, fatigue, depression, breast tenderness and food cravings. Most multivitamins contain sufficient vitamin B6. Good food sources for B6 include fish, poultry, grains, sweet potatoes, avocados, soy-based meat substitutes and bananas.

## OMEGA-3 FATTY ACIDS

Remember the cold water fish from the Mediterranean Diet? They're chock full of omega-3 fatty acids, an essential nutrient. Essential nutrients are necessary for good physical and mental health, but are not made by the body. Recent studies suggest that omega-3 can boost the immune system, alleviate depression, and reduce inflammation and joint pain.

## AMINO ACIDS

Amino acids are the building blocks of skin, hair, bones, muscles and hormones, but half the amino acids we need aren't manufactured by the body. Instead, we get them from supplements and good nutrition. Tyrosine, tryptophan and gamma aminobutyric acid (GABA) all influence mood and have a positive, calming effect. A cup of cottage cheese or low-fat yogurt each day contains the tyrosine your body needs, while five ounces of turkey breast or

salmon will cover your tryptophan intake. GABA is found in several food sources, with the highest concentrations in fish and wheat bran.

## Random Vitamin Trivia

On Jan. 1, 1996, Betty Rubble first appeared as a Flintstone vitamin, 27 years after her series co-stars. What's up with that?

## Herbal Remedies

For the last 20 years, Americans have been using herbal remedies in record numbers. Herbal preparations come from the leaves, roots, seeds, bark, fruit and/or stems of plants and have been used for millennia by women around the world to treat headaches, cramps, anxiety and more. They are not regulated by the FDA so the purity and concentration of active ingredients in a single dose can vary among different brands of the same herb. If you find one that works for you, stick with it. As with most things, buyer beware: Many companies have jumped on the herbal bandwagon, making outrageous and unproven claims about their magic potions. Remember, there's no miracle cure for PMS, so if it sounds too good to be true, it probably is.

Herbal remedies are great, but don't get carried away. Herbal or not, many of these remedies can be quite strong. Stay away from anything that contains ma huang, yohimbe, stephania, chaparral, comfrey, jin bu huan, lobelia, magnolia, willow bark or germander. The FDA has concluded that these herbs may cause health problems more serious than the worst PMS.

## Extra Rx

Besides understanding the behavior modifications and remedies that facilitate PMS improvement, women should recognize what exacerbates their symptoms. We've listed just a few common irritants; feel free to add your own.

* Miss America® Pageants
* Anything Star Wars®
* Paris Hilton
* Mouth breathers
* People who use the phrase, "That's what I'm talking about!"
* Man purses

## CHASTEBERRY

Chasteberry is the "go to" remedy for PMS. This shrub can help mood swings, anger, headaches, breast tenderness and swelling. German scientists found that women taking 20 mg of chasteberry reported a 52% reduction in PMS symptoms. If you're on the pill or hormone replacement therapies, check with your doctor before taking chasteberry.

## DONG QUAI

Dong quai has been used in Asia for centuries to treat symptoms of menopause and perimenopause, but may also be helpful in treating hormone imbalances during PMS. The secret to dong quai's success is that it corrects the body's hormone balance. It's available as a powdered root, capsule, extract or tea and can be particularly useful in conjunction with acupuncture. Skip dong quai entirely during your period as it can intensify bleeding.

## EVENING PRIMROSE OIL

Evening primrose oil alleviates breast tenderness, depression, irritability and fluid retention. The oil is available in capsules and is best absorbed when taken with a B-complex vitamin and vitamin C. To avoid stomach problems, take evening primrose oil capsules after eating.

## ST. JOHN'S WORT

St. John's Wort is a natural alternative to prescription anti-depressants and helps to combat the PMS blues. If you're taking prescription anti-depressant or anti-anxiety medication, check with your doctor before trying St. John's Wort.

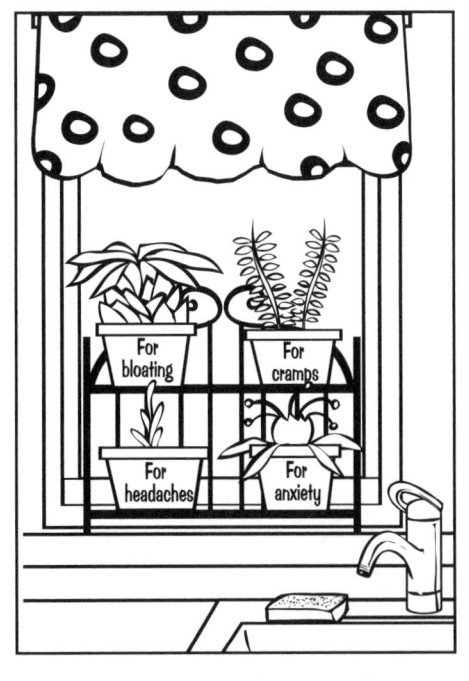

The PMS Window Garden

## VALERIAN ROOT

Valerian Root has been used for 1,000 years to reduce anxiety, tension and insomnia without being addictive. An added benefit is that it doesn't cause the morning grogginess common to many prescription sleep aids. However, it should never be used with other sedatives, tranquilizers or any anti-depressants. A word to the wise: This is one of the smelliest herbal remedies, so stick with pills, capsules or teas and avoid extracts.

# Hot Stuff

A study regarding women's attraction to the opposite sex during PMS was conducted recently by a renowned department of psychology. It revealed that the kind of male face a woman finds attractive can differ depending on where she is in her menstrual cycle. For instance, if ovulating, women are drawn to men with rugged, masculine features. However, during PMS, a woman is likely to be attracted to a man with a knitting needle lodged in his temple and a TV remote jammed up his butt while he's on fire.

# How About Some Sex with Your Vitamins?

It may or may not be common knowledge that orgasm relieves menstrual cramps and stress (see more in "Choose Pleasure Over Pain" on page 109) but it's definitely the most pleasurable treatment; worst case scenario, it might take your mind off your problems for a few glorious minutes! However, if you're one of the many women who lose their sex drive during PMS, it's possible that with relief from your other symptoms, your libido will return to normal. If not, there are herbal preparations that might help.

### DAMIANA

A South American herb often cited for its anti-depressant and aphrodisiac effects, Damiana has been known to break the cycle of depression and kick start a woman's sex drive. Not depressed? It could still do wonders for your libido with some studies suggesting that Damiana functions like testosterone, the hormone of desire in men and women. Try the recommended dose and then tighten the bolts in your chandelier!

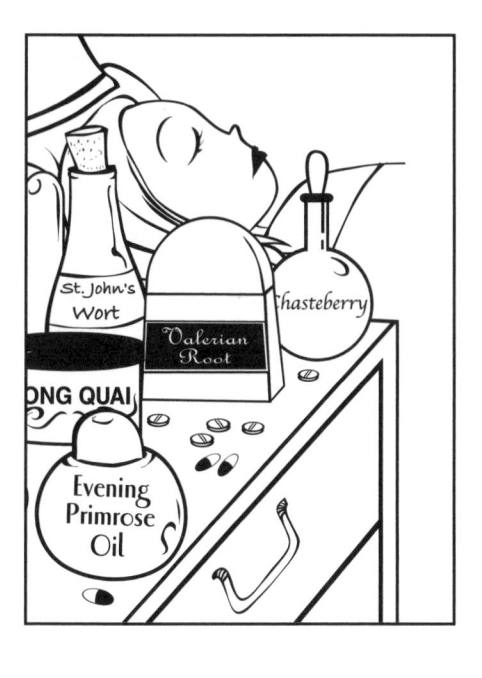

## TANGO

An herbal mixture based on an ancient Chinese formula, Tango contains chrysanthemum flowers, three types of mushrooms, ginseng, cinnamon and licorice. Both men and women cite an increase in sexual desire and pleasure, as well as easier, longer and stronger orgasms with Tango. Share it with someone you love – quickly! It's usually taken an hour or so before sex, or daily for an energy boost.

# Crash Course: Hormones 101

## Hyla Cass, M.D.
### Specialist in integrative medicine and psychiatry

Our mothers once called them "women's problems." Now we know that these mood swings and physical changes, from PMS to menopause, are all part of a delicate balance among our hormones. In my years of practicing integrative medicine, I have helped hundreds of women overcome PMS and menopausal symptoms naturally.

The cycles of the main female sex hormones, estrogen and progesterone, have powerful effects on our wellbeing and are intimately connected to the chemical mediators of mood, our neurotransmitters. Any variation in one affects the

other; for example, a dip in estrogen will lower the feel-good neurotransmitter, serotonin, and insufficient progesterone will prevent GABA, the calming neurotransmitter, from doing its job.

All women have the same hormones but in varying quantities, making your hormonal profile as unique as your fingerprint. When your hormones are in harmony, you will have predictable menstrual cycles and moods. When out of balance, your hormones will cause irregular cycles and a host of PMS symptoms.

# Medical Management

For a full picture of your hormonal status you need to check levels of estrogen, progesterone, DHEA-S, testosterone and pregnenolone in blood, saliva or urine. For perimenopausal women, FSH (follicle-stimulating hormone) and LH (luteinizing hormone) tests assess ovarian function.

If you'd like to try home testing with kits available online, take these tests on days 19-21 of your cycle, with day 1 being the first day of your period. If you are menopausal, it won't matter when you take the tests. If you're irregular, do your best to estimate the appropriate time.

## Hormone Therapy

If testing reveals that your hormone levels are below the normal range, it may be due to perimenopause or other physiological factors. Faced with fluctuating hormones, doctors have traditionally prescribed synthetic hormone replacement therapy (HRT), such as Premarin® and Prempro® to correct imbalances. The latest data indicate that synthetic hormones may increase the risk of breast cancer, so they should be used at the lowest effective dose for the shortest possible time. There are other

ways to balance hormones successfully, ranging from using supplements and herbs to bio-identical hormone therapy (see the following section).

# Natural Ways to Balance Sex Hormones

There are specific supplements for PMS, such as magnesium, borage oil, and B vitamins, especially B6 and folic acid. Herbal remedies include dong quai, chasteberry, and wild yam extract. These can all be found in formulations like PMS Balance. I have had many women report almost immediate relief upon taking this or a similar formula, while other women may take a month or two to feel the full effects.

When these supplements are not enough, I prescribe bio-identical hormones. Made from highly purified derivatives of soy and wild yams, they are carbon copies of your own natural hormones. Bio-identical hormones are available only from compounding pharmacies, and are prescribed by your doctor based on your individual hormonal needs determined by your lab tests. You can also use over-the-counter natural progesterone cream.

As I say to my patients over and over again, "You don't have to live with PMS." With the help of bio-identical hormones and supplements, PMS has truly become a thing of the past for many women and their loved ones.

*Suggestions for men who have to address women
during those perilous periods:*

*RISKY - What's for dinner?*
*SAFER - Where do you want to go for dinner?*
*SAFEST - What should I clean the toilets with?*

*RISKY - Are you wearing that?*
*SAFER - Those sweats accentuate your beautiful eyes.*
*SAFEST - What should I clean the toilets with?*

*RISKY - Should you be eating that?*
*SAFER - Can I get you a glass of wine with that?*
*SAFEST - What should I clean the toilets with?*

*RISKY - What did you do all day?*
*SAFER - I hope you didn't work too hard today!*
*SAFEST - What should I clean the toilets with?*

# Love Me Tender... and Bloated

Men, no matter how sensitive or evolved, just don't get PMS —
literally or figuratively. But, imagine if PMS were a dual-gender
offender. What if Michael Jordan had provoked the nation's
curiosity with "wings or without?" instead of "boxers or briefs?"
Or, if Dan Marino had cited sensitive nipples and low testosterone
as explanations for an "off" game every month or so?

No doubt, males undergo hormonal changes – maybe they've experienced acne or a few regrettable "keep the lights off" one-night stands as young adults – but they've never endured the persistent physical and lightning-quick emotional changes that women feel. If only Lance Armstrong had copped to the agony of water retention in spandex shorts, then maybe, just maybe, understanding PMS would be a priority for men.

## Bewildered Bedfellows

PMS affects everyone who crosses your path. Husbands, lovers, children and the pizza delivery man all bear the brunt of your distress. With 50% of women reporting PMS at some point in their lives, sooner or later a mother, sister, girlfriend or coworker will introduce men to its wild ride. Sure, men can rattle off a few "on the rag" jokes or mumble something snide at the first telltale premenstrual sign, but if we don't educate them, they usually add fuel to the already raging hormonal fire. Even well-meaning mates don't know what to do or say and it's likely that whatever they try will just set us off...again.

Women wish men would try harder to understand, and it's tough to fathom why they don't. Researchers at the University of Washington found that 75% of men reported that their lives were moderately to greatly disrupted by their partners' PMS. However, instead of finding constructive or helpful ways of dealing with the symptoms, most men respond by expressing anger or withdrawing.

Are women with PMS really that scary? The answer is a resounding "could be." Their monthly split personalities have been known to terrify guys. It's a male cultural thing, related to long-held ideas about how women should act. Men may not even be aware that they hold these beliefs but society has slowly shaped their thinking

over the course of their lives (Playboy®... Penthouse®... Big-Jugged Bootylicious Mamas. Just one theory.)

It's no secret that men aren't as comfortable with feelings as women. Most men would rather take phone calls from their mothers-in-law than field questions such as, "Do you love me?" "What are you thinking?" and the dreaded, "Do you think she's prettier than me?" If it's a "PMSing" woman who's asking those loaded questions, then "Welcome to hell!" is all he'll hear anyway.

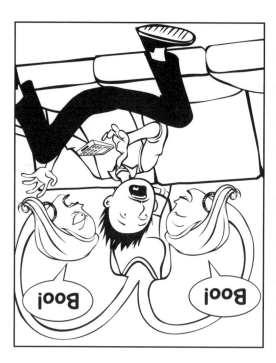

## WomanSpeak

Speaking of what he hears, try to remember that men are simple creatures, accustomed to all-purpose grunts and shrugs. We, on the other hand, have a language all our own. Every woman knows that it's a rare (and usually gay) man who has the girl-talk decoder ring.

What we say isn't necessarily what we mean – especially during PMS. Admit it. When you ask your plaid-clad, backward-cap donning man-child "Are you wearing that?" what you really mean

is "You've got to be kidding!" Or, when loverboy proposes a trip to visit his parents instead of your annual beach vacation and you say "I'll think about it," we'll bet dollars to the hidden donuts in your underwear drawer that what you really mean is "Not a chance in hell!" Men who haven't figured this out yet are simply doomed!

More than anything else – particularly during PMS – we want to be understood by our guys. To avoid the lines of communication getting crossed, try to keep responses short, simple and honest, such as "yes," "no" or "bite me." In the meantime, we've included some translations for men on page 41 on the other side of this book, which should clue them in until they learn the language or you drop the double-talk.

## Please Make Sense!

For most of us, when PMS hits, our well-honed communication skills and shaving habits beat a hasty retreat. We become snappish, angry or even funny in a scary way (or is it scary in a funny way?) as simmering feelings finally boil over; other times, neediness or weepiness descends like a dense fog. Both the physical and emotional symptoms we experience can start a chain reaction in all intimate relationships. Everyone's angry, hurt and confused. And 'round, and 'round it goes.

Both men and women claim that the other uses PMS as an excuse for relationship problems. Husbands believe that wives cite it as a reason for not having sex or behaving irrationally, and wives think their husbands use it as an excuse to take an emotional vacation and pay less attention to them. Over time, as the months and years of living with PMS take their toll, couples become more defensive and destructive communication patterns take hold. We stop listening to each other, believing we already know what the other has to say. Love and respect are buried under the rubble of unresolved conflicts, cramps and candy wrappers.

In some relationships, women describe feeling a total lack of love and affection for their partner during **PMS**. A week later, when their period begins, those same women fall in love again, and buy out every card in Hallmark's® "I'm Sorry, Temporary Insanity" line.

The effect this has on our partners can be overwhelming. Remember, your significant other can't read your mind. He can only respond to what you say and your body language, which can be brutal during **PMS**. Accordingly, while you may assume all is forgiven once the tide changes (and flows), your significant other might take longer to get over his hurt feelings, and possibly his fear of you!

# Irritable Male Syndrome

British researchers may have come up with an explanation for why men get grumpy and temperamental. The newly minted Irritable Male Syndrome (IMS) could explain aggression, male moodiness and depression after football season. Apparently, men of any age who suffer stress can experience sudden dips in testosterone, making them bad-tempered, nervous or weepy. One suggestion is that testosterone replacement therapy may restore men to their "normal" state.

Other male "syndromes" that we'd like to propose to the American Medical Association:

* Hands in Pants Syndrome
* Habitual Gas Disorder
* After-Sex Narcolepsy
* Socks & Sandals Blindness
* Inability to Write Legibly Affliction

# The Battle of the Sexes

The happiest home can turn into a hellish one if family members aren't on the same **PMS** page. Whether your relationship is strewn with sexual landmines or it always comes down to a war over whose turn it is to vacuum, these are the high-risk situations that send you and your not-always beloved into a tailspin. The first step is to identify the sources of stress and anger in your relationships. By anticipating those triggers, you can work to defuse them in advance, before PMS sinks its sharp teeth into you and your loved ones.

Is Wednesday the night to take out the garbage? If so, this simple task may become the focus of a fight. Is Saturday "date night" with your honey? Be aware that sex might be anticipated by one of you, but not the other. You can avoid the dicey situations entirely (it takes a lot less energy to drag the trash can to the curb than to fight over it for an hour) or come up with an alternate plan in advance ("Let's reschedule date night so we can both enjoy it."). Use the communication tools below to get what you need before a small problem turns into a Jerry Springer episode.

# Loose Lips Sink Relationships

Remember that men, by nature, want to fix things. If you came with instructions or a screwdriver, they'd fix your **PMS** in a heartbeat, but you're not a toaster. To help them, you have to describe your **PMS** in terms of what you want from them. When you're direct, you say exactly what you feel and need (i.e. "I feel like I need diamonds...and Fritos®"). In the process, you remove an enormous burden from the people who love you and have been wracking their brains trying to figure out what to do

about the unpredictable stranger at the dinner table. Being direct means no sarcasm, hostility, aggression or defensiveness. It means speaking honestly *and listening*, and it works with everyone.

In the following example, our PMS mom is frustrated because her husband keeps the kids up past their bedtime. She's with them all day and needs some quiet time to herself, especially during PMS. She's carefully avoiding "you" statements like, "You get the kids excited and it takes hours to get them to sleep" or "You're making it extra hard for me to work on my PMS." Instead, she's making "I" statements, focusing on what she needs and how it will help.

To communicate effectively, start with a little planning. Schedule a time to discuss the issue, but not during PMS:

> ✳ I'll ask Tom if he's willing to talk about this tomorrow. If that doesn't work for him, we'll schedule a conversation this weekend.

When you've scheduled a time to discuss it, describe the problem and how you feel about it using "I" not "you" statements:

> ✳ "I feel frustrated and hurt when the schedule gets disrupted. It undermines my authority with the kids and makes it tough for me to have the alone time I need."

Ask for what you want simply:

> ✳ "I'd like to stick to a bedtime and I really need your help enforcing it."

Reinforce the chances of getting what you want by describing a positive outcome:

> ✳ "If the kids stick to their schedule, I'll have time to focus on my PMS recovery plan and I'll get better faster. If there's something you need from me, I'd be happy to help."

Speak clearly, maintain eye contact and avoid taking a whiny or accusatory tone. If you find that the conversation is not going well, suggest that you take a break. That will stop "automatic" aggressive responses long enough for both of you to consider constructive alternatives.

If this method of communication is new for you, it can help to practice your requests in front of a mirror. Watch your body language and facial expressions. (Note: If your mouth is foaming or your head is spinning like Regan's in the *Exorcist*, schedule extra practice time.) Listen to your tone to ensure that it's calm and even. Anticipate objections in advance and plan responses to them that don't include the phrases "Payback is a bitch!" and/or "Burn in hell!"

At the right time, you can explain to your partner what you're doing to get PMS out of both of your lives for good. You might talk about food choices, supplements, exercise and the other strategies that you're using to send your premenstrual princess packing. Before you know it, you'll be communicating like a pro and getting what you need to feel better.

# Lighten Up

Don't forget to schedule some lighthearted time together; see a funny movie or go to a comedy club. Laughter is the glue that binds good relationships, releasing tension and keeping speaker and listener emotionally attuned. It can establish, or restore, a positive emotional climate between two people and is an invaluable tool when PMS causes some pretty awkward moments. For more on creating a PMS partnership that works, read "Getting Well, Together" on page 129.

# Don't Kid the Kids

One of the most common reasons that women with **PMS** seek help is that they fear what their symptoms might be doing to their children. Successful parenting requires consistency, but it's tough to be consistent when you end up bribing your little ones with candy or extra TV time for a few minutes of peace and quiet on your worst days.

Kids of all ages just want to feel secure in your love for them, so the slightest behavioral changes or mood shifts in their parents, especially their mothers, may cause confusion. Usually, that confusion translates to anxiety and neediness, and it's extra tough to deal with a clingy child when all you want is to be left alone.

Rather than telling young children that you have an illness that recurs monthly, a pretty scary thought for them, it's safer to

describe your needs and your behavior. For example, "Mommy has a tummy ache and needs to rest for a little while" is much more reassuring than "Let me die in peace." Or, "If I seem angry at you sometimes, it's not because I don't love you, it's because I'm not feeling my best. I'll feel better in a couple of days, but I need your cooperation." Most importantly, make sure your kids know that they're not the cause of your problems.

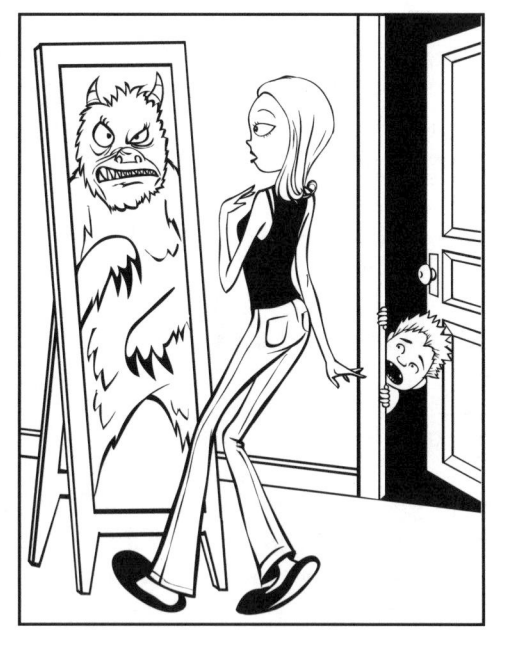

# Truth or Consequences

The idea that everyone will be happy if you can only get rid of your PMS is wishful thinking. Couples and families have underlying tensions that have nothing to do with PMS, though symptoms may amplify any conflicts. Perhaps you and your family have been blaming your PMS for problems that aren't yours at all.

In some families, there may be lingering emotions that continue to affect everyone after PMS is long gone. With some time and consistent effort, this PMS hangover should subside. In other households, the absence of PMS may make it clear that there are additional problems that need to be resolved for the family to become functional and whole. On the bright side, issues will be easier to cope with and work on without that premenstrual time bomb hanging over everyone's heads.

Couples often take a "second honeymoon" or vacation to work out their problems. Remember that even without the daily stressors of family life, you're still taking your troubles with you. Family or couple's counseling is often the best solution. The unique perspective of someone without an agenda or an axe to grind (or bury in your head) can breathe new life into a relationship. Psychologists, licensed clinical social workers (LCSWs), rabbis, pastors or priests can all provide assistance when you're not sure where to turn.

# Complain in Composition

One great coping tool for PMS casualties is to keep a journal. You can tell your journal absolutely anything and it won't criticize, blame or take away your Froot Loops®. Writing down your feelings, rather than blurting them out, gives you the

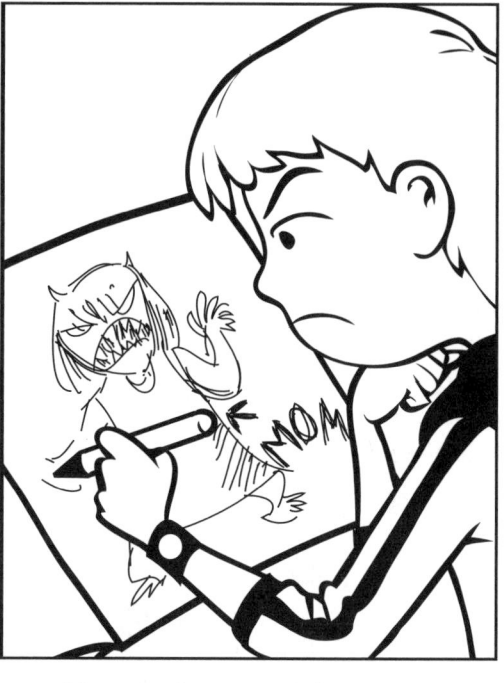

chance to review them later on to decide if they're rooted in reality or premenstrual misery. If they're real, you can discuss them in a diplomatic fashion when you're calm and able to bring some perspective to the conversation – as opposed to nunchucks.

Journal writing is a wonderful lifelong habit that encourages creativity, healthy introspection and stress reduction. If you have children who are old enough, you might encourage them to do the same. It's also a great way to carve out some quiet time for yourself as everyone goes to their own rooms to write their thoughts, doodle or draw pictures of mommy with her second, fire-breathing head.

# The Single Sufferer

If you're single and searching, here's a helpful hint: Never go on a first date during PMS. It's probably best to hold off until you are back to your fabulous and dateable self. You want to give any potential partner the chance to know and like you without PMS pushing his "NEXT!" button. An online dating site, JDate®, counsels women not to discuss their weight, past boyfriends, divorces or money until well into the relationship. Add PMS

(and meddlesome parents) to that list. After all, do you want to hear about his ongoing battle with athlete's foot on your first date?

Whether you're actively looking for "the one" or satisfied with your solo status, take time to plan a red-letter day. After all, PMS is – for good or bad – a distinction of womanhood. While women in relationships want to hide out in a cave during PMS, single women often feel lonely or isolated. Combat that loneliness by treating yourself to a night at the movies (avoid the tearjerkers) or schedule time with a friend. You may have more freedom to work on your recovery plan and indulge in soothing self-care than your married counterparts. Celebrate by donning a red shirt or bandanna and doing whatever you please, short of eating your weight in Oreos®, to make yourself feel good.

## Party with Your PMS

No matter what your dating status, round up your girlfriends and invite them over for an evening of pampering and amusement. Clear the house of men, specify a "sweats-only" dress code and settle in for a night of female bonding. Watch chick flicks, discuss the most popular self-help books, or give each other manicures and pedicures. Share your most memorable PMS horror stories or hilarious anecdotes. Everyone can bitch guilt-free because all partygoers are, or have been, in the same bloated boat. A fitting way to end the party is with a piñata. Each woman takes a turn whacking the sugar-free-candy-filled, papier maché patsy. It's a great stress reliever!

While you might want to take the advice in this book seriously, don't take yourself too seriously. Make time to watch a favorite sitcom, joke with friends, read the funnies, or have a good giggle at nature's best comics: children and animals. It's nearly impossible to stay miserable or mad when you're laughing!

# Me, Myself & PMS

Although it's ideal to get everyone onboard, your family and friends may or may not be instrumental in your **PMS** recovery plan. Ultimately, what matters most is your own commitment to health and healing. **PMS** can deal a heavy blow to your self-esteem, but setting small, manageable goals and then accomplishing them can rebuild your confidence quickly.

Your other relationships will be most successful when you feel good about who you are and what you're doing. Take baby steps and the time to nurture hope and practice self-care. At the end of the day, the most important relationship you have is with yourself.

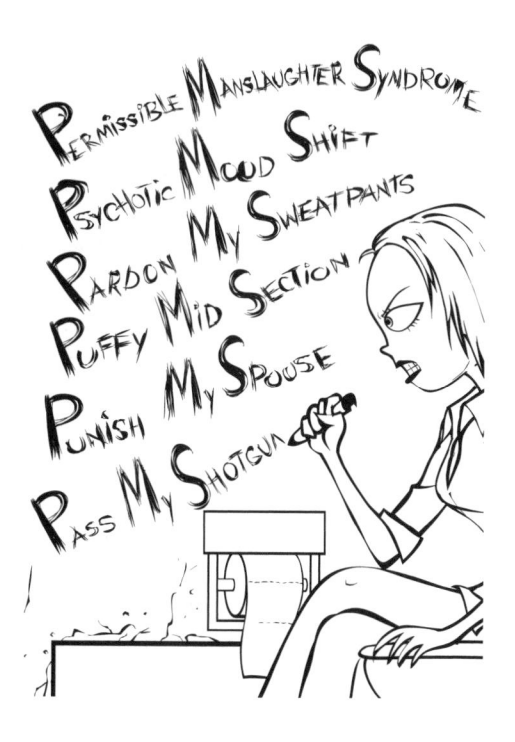

Permissible Manslaughter Syndrome

Psychotic Mood Shift

Pardon My Sweatpants

Puffy Mid Section

Punish My Spouse

Pass My Shotgun

# On the Job With PMS

## (Don't Get Worked Up!)

Sometimes all it takes is one chauvinistic bozo by the water cooler to blow the top off your premenstrual volcano. Even with the best intentions, it's not easy to put your mother or PMS symptoms on hold at work. You can only keep things under wraps for so long before your tolerance threshold has been trampled and you're wondering, *Why didn't I just didn't call in sick?*

# Getting Down to Business — or Not!

According to recent estimates, menstrual misfortunes cost U.S. industry eight percent of its total wages in lost productivity and sick days. Women usually cite cramps and premenstrual migraines (and a good clearance sale – be honest!) as reasons to stay home. Other PMS woes are rarely considered a good enough reason to be absent; instead, we go to work with our caustic tempers in tow, giving ourselves a bad name.

Most of us have miserable and even occasionally humiliating premenstrual and menstrual workday tales we'd like to forget – including ruining luxury light-colored fabrics and summoning a relative or close friend to bring a change of clothes and an industrial-sized bottle of ibuprofen. However, as humbling as those scenarios may be, they usually don't make international headlines. Consider Russian astronaut Valentina Tereshkova: In 1973, she had to return to earth after only three days in space when she got her period in zero gravity!

Perhaps we should take a tip from our female friends in Argentina, where the constitution permits women to take days off if they have menstrual problems. In India, women are excused from housework and cooking, as it's believed that any food they prepare may be spoiled by their menstrual blood. We're willing to bet that rumor was started by one clever woman!

## Time Out

In the U.S., there's been chit-chat in the legislature about declaring PMS a disability, and a few companies have proposed days off for women with PMS or difficult periods. If businesses were to grant excused absences for PMS, one could only imagine the possibilities: "Leave-Me-Alone Leave," "Decompress Days," or "Bitch Itch."

# Thar She Blows!

There's no doubt that problems at work increase the severity of PMS. Restrained, professional and even civil communication can be a tall order when you're suffering from physical and emotional symptoms – and heads look like an invitation to batting practice!

Women often report increased sensitivity to noise, making the usual office buzz an unbearable distraction. Hypersensitivity to odors can also be a concern making the coworker with grooming issues in the next cubicle a menses minefield. Other women are persistently cold or hot during PMS, and find their office environments unpleasantly arctic or tropical for a week or two a month. Finally, for those whose self-esteem is affected, whether by premenstrual weight gain or anxiety, even constructive criticism from fellow employees or supervisors can be tough to take.

When we feel lousy about ourselves, it colors how we view the world and we become thin-skinned to the opinions of others. One successful woman, after hearing that her latest work wasn't up to par, locked herself in her office and spent the day turning every piece of paper into confetti. She's not crazy and she's still employed, but her PMS made her act irrationally. Two days later, she was back at work, printing out all the documents she shredded and filing them. She got help, but regrets not taking charge of her PMS sooner...and laminating her work!

# Making it Work at Work

You have your work cut out for you if your place of business is within a male-dominated industry, and there are still plenty of them. Dealing with PMS can be especially tough when surrounded by gentlemen who aren't so gentlemanly; insensitive and ill-timed

jokes about wives or girlfriends and "that time of month" are hard to take. After all, most of us don't have much of a sense of humor when we're achy, swollen and seething!

Working in these environments, we feel extra pressure to cope with and overcome PMS to avoid being labeled as irrational, ineffective or weak – as in the proverbial "weaker sex." It can be tough to keep up the perception that you're one of the guys, when truthfully, you're not.

## Comebacks for Women with PMS and Insensitive Coworkers!

(We don't recommend trying them with the boss.)

* Is it time for your medication or mine?
* My bloated belly will be gone in a few days. What about yours?
* I'm not cranky. I'm just in a bad mood when you're around.

So, how should you handle your PMS in the workplace? Women's magazines have long counseled readers to tell their bosses and coworkers that they have PMS. That's a personal choice. We've fought long and hard for the same rights and pay as men and all it takes is one Neanderthal male boss – or worse, a PMS-free unsympathetic female superior – to use our symptoms against us. On the other puffy hand, comments about how employees of a particular gender are not suited for certain jobs, or a pattern of statements about employee conduct such as "She probably has PMS," violate your civil rights. Of course, no one wants to do battle in court, so carefully weigh the potential risks and personalities you're dealing with when considering if or how to divulge your PMS.

# PMS Red Flags

While you're working on your PMS, cut colleagues a break and warn them to approach at their own risk. Websites like www.pmscentral.com offer cute desktop flags that will announce your woes to the world. Emblazoned with "PMS Danger Zone," these flags will keep annoying coworkers at bay. We can almost hear you singing, "I am woman, hear me ROAR!"

# 9 to 5 Coping Techniques

Whether you choose to announce your PMS with a red flag or keep it to your irritated self, there will be days when you have to deal at work. Assuming you've been refining your chow choices, stepping up the physical activity and supplementing with supplements, what else can you do while you're waiting for your symptoms to improve?

First, take a good look at your environment. What changes would make it more comfortable other than flinging the motivational posters and a few associates out the window? Asking for an ergonomic chair or buying one for yourself can make a huge difference not only to the aches and pains of PMS, but also to your mood and general productivity. These chairs can be pricey, but will repay your investment with improved posture, better circulation, fewer back and neck problems, and a decreased chance of developing spider veins on your legs.

Try the new generation of support hose that massage your legs, improve circulation and help your energy level all day long. You can also pack a traditional heating pad or one of the new, disposable, air-activated heating pads in your briefcase to help with cramps or back pain.

Next, invest in some earplugs, the small squishy ones that go into the outer ear canal. You probably can't wear them all day, but you may be able to give yourself some blessed moments of peace and quiet, whether at lunch, on bathroom breaks or if you're discreet, in Monday morning meetings. It's amazing how much restorative power a few minutes of silence can have, particularly with some deep breathing and neck rolls. For more about stretches and relaxation techniques, see "PMS: A License to Chill" on page 101.

Enlist a coworker to walk with you before work or during lunch to support your exercise program. Be sure to stock your desk drawer with some sugar-free chocolate, herbal tea, raw almonds or any other healthy snack foods to get you through the tough days.

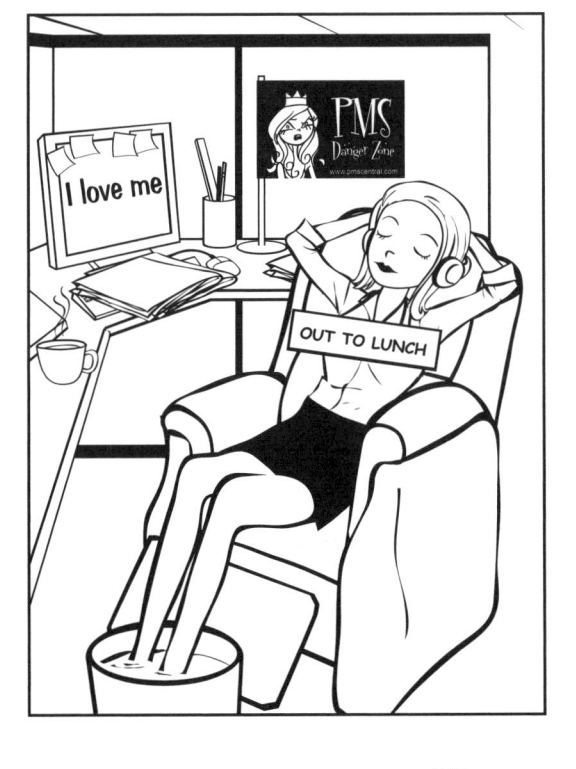

Finally, keep some reinforcements nearby to soothe and promote self-care: a rich hand cream for a quickie massage, a good cover-up for PMS break-outs, your favorite lipstick for a self-esteem boost and a CD or MP3 player loaded with your favorite tunes for a pick-me-up. You can take care of yourself and your work responsibilities at the same time; it just takes a little forethought.

## Take-Home Tips

Consider holding seminars to educate your male coworkers on the finer points of behaving around women with PMS. ALL the females in their lives will thank you. Some suggestions include:

* Gift Giving 101
* Just say, "Yes, dear." (pre-requisite: It's Not All About You)
* There's Only One Answer to "Do I Look Fat?", parts 1 & 2
* Advanced Ice Tray Filling (pre-requisite: Toilet Paper Roll Replacing)
* Shut Up and Fix It! (marriage 1, marriage 2, marriage 3 levels)

## Plan When You Can

You've been tracking your cycle and your symptoms, so you know when your PMS pod pal is likely to appear. (You can also use a website like www.pmscentral.com that will email you with a PMS reminder so you can send up a flare.) If you're lucky enough to work for a company that believes in the eighth wonder of the world, flex-time, you've got it made. You can work around your PMS, and accumulate enough hours to take time off on your worst days. Lately, more companies are making that option available to employees.

If you're able to telecommute – work from home – then you have the best of all possible situations. You can get down to business in your jammies, take breaks when needed, and you don't have the additional pressure of pretending you're just fine when you feel like something that crawled out from under a rock.

Whatever your situation, try to schedule important meetings, presentations, projects, lunch with the boss, or travel around

your PMS until you get it reliably under control...for everyone's sake. If you're working as part of a team or don't have the independence of setting your own schedule, you can still accommodate your symptoms. For example, if you know that a project deadline conflicts with your PMS, put in extra work ahead of time so that when you're feeling bad, the majority is already done. There are ways to work it out at work!

# By the Light of the Moon

Studies have shown women who work the night shift frequently have more severe PMS symptoms. The body's clock lives in the hypothalamus, the same part of the brain that regulates your menstrual cycle, and it's easily upset. If you find yourself jet-setting across time zones or staying up all night working, you might have to kiss your predictable menstrual cycle goodbye for a month or two.

# Office Support

Another way to wage war against PMS is to speak – or vent – to people who sympathize with your efforts. It's important to have a little support, other than undergarments. Studies have consistently found that social support can decrease the effects of stress and illness, while boosting self-esteem.

Significant others are wonderful, but they may have their own issues with your PMS. Another option is to look for a local PMS support group. Try women's Internet sites, such as health.yahoo.com/groups, or get in touch with a community center or women's health clinic. The idea of being in a room with other women who feel as lousy as you do may be horrifying, but the chances of everyone having PMS at the same time are slim. Fellow sufferers can cheer on your recovery, share their own

experiences and techniques for mastering the misery and compare the advantages of elastic-waist attire.

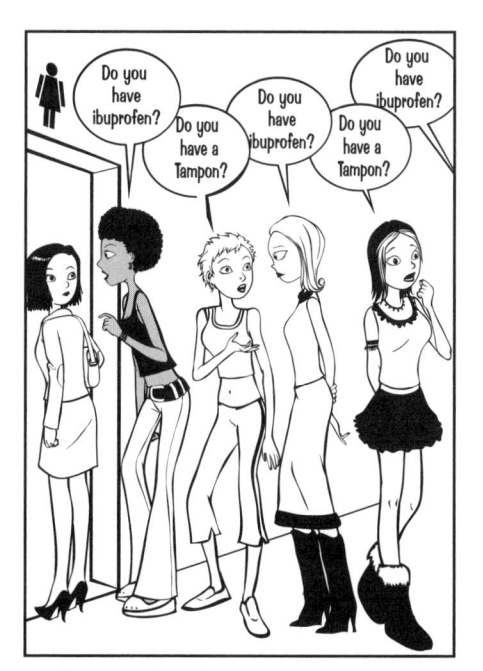

## Girl Power

Whether you join a group, form your own or find a friend to help you stick to your PMS plan, the motivation and support can be invaluable. A recent UCLA study has unearthed some proof that women form special and therapeutic bonds. Whereas men tend to fight or flee when stressed, we release a hormone, oxytocin, that buffers the fight or flight instinct and encourages us to nurture or gather with other women and host sex toy parties. The more we do this, the more stuff we collect that we never use, but more notably, the more oxytocin is released, which further calms us. It's evolution's alternative to a hot bubble bath and a book with Fabio on the cover.

Our families are the cornerstones of our lives, but friends are critical to our good health. Research confirms that the more friends we have, the less likely we are to develop physical problems as we age and the more likely we are to lead happy lives. The results are so significant that not having close friends or confidantes is as detrimental to our health as obesity or smoking. So, put down that chili cheese dog, snuff out that butt and make a friend!

*How many women with PMS does it take to screw in a light bulb?*

*ONE! And do you know WHY it only takes one? Because NO ONE else in this damn house knows how to change a light bulb! They wouldn't even realize the bulb burned out. They'd sit in the dark for a week before they'd notice. And, even IF they did notice, they WOULDN'T BE ABLE TO FIND THE LIGHT BULBS without my help! But if they managed to miraculously find the light bulbs, the chair they'd drag over to stand on to change the stupid light bulb would be left there until I DRAGGED IT BACK! And, the box that the frickin' light bulbs came in would be left there, too. WHY? Because NO ONE besides me ever TAKES OUT THE GARBAGE!! It's a miracle we haven't all been buried alive under the garbage throughout the house. The house! It would take an army to clean this...I'm sorry...what was the question?*

# PMS: A License to Chill

Ask most women to rank the order in which their needs and those of their loved ones are met, and they'll tell you they come somewhere after the family pet and just ahead of houseplants. The worst part is that it may be their fault!

We're accustomed to putting others' needs ahead of our own. First, we take care of parents, grandparents, spouses, children, friends and even bosses; then, if there's any time or energy left, we attend to ourselves. Guess what? In the long run, that just doesn't work. Like everyone else, we need to nurture our dreams, creativity, bodies and minds. If we don't, we're giving everyone, especially ourselves, less than our best.

# PMS Rhymes with Stress

PMS maims, but stress kills. A quick Internet search on the effects of stress yields endless articles about everything from infertility, high blood pressure and cancer to headaches and excessive retail shopping. Stress is an unconscious and automatic reaction to anything we believe may be threatening to us.

Except when we're watching Antonio Banderas films, never does the mind-body connection speak louder than when we're under stress. Whether we are confronted by imminent danger or the town blabbermouth in a checkout line, the results are the same. Up goes our heart rate, blood pressure and adrenaline production, and down goes blood flow to the extremities, our digestive function, immune system activity and bullcrap tolerance.

Theoretically, this reaction subsides once the situation has resolved, allowing our bodies to return to normal. However, women who are frequently under stress, whether from PMS or the balding men with razor-sharp toenails lying beside them, tend to stay locked into a pattern of stress response. If your shoulders are hunched up somewhere around your earlobes, you're one of those women.

# Time Is Money

While many of us can apply mascara, peel a banana, scold a child, consult a map and juggle a cell phone between our ear and shoulder while driving in rush hour traffic, most of us aren't very good at time management and prioritizing. There are days when everything seems urgent. The best solution is to treat time like money – in truth, it's far more precious – and think ahead about how you're going to spend it.

# Lighten Your (Mental) Load

If you have perfectionist tendencies, try to get a little perspective and have a chuckle at your own expense. For instance, remind yourself that when people drop by, they've come to see you, not your flawless makeup or dust-free corners. So, stop doing things over and over again to make them just right; instead, cross them off the list and move on.

You might need to set limits at home and work. Figure out what you can really do. There are only so many hours in the day. Establish boundaries with yourself and others. Don't be afraid to say no to requests for your time and energy, otherwise, you'll spread yourself too thin and not be of much use to anyone.

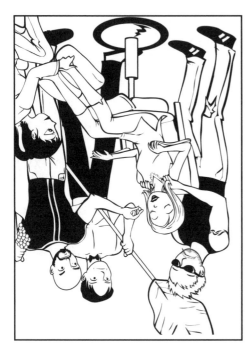

No matter how busy you are, set aside at least 15 to 30 minutes each day to do something that's just for you. Catch up with an old friend on the phone, read the tabloids, get a facial or listen to a favorite CD. Treat the things you do for yourself, like relaxation or exercise, as if they were appointments with VIPs. Would you show up late for an important client? Would you stand up your best friend? No way!

# Kick the Doubters to the Curb

One of the nicest things we can do for ourselves is to remove as many negative influences from our lives as possible. Along with giving PMS the boot, it's time to take a good, honest look at the people, places and things in your life. Is there a friend who's negative all the time or relentlessly self-absorbed, and drains you of your already depleted energy? If so, it might be time to say, "Buh bye!" Does your doctor really listen to you and take your problems seriously? If not, find a healthcare practitioner who gives you and your PMS the time of day. Is a coworker making your life miserable? Schedule a heart-to-heart, based on the communication principles on page 83.

Of course, we can't rid ourselves of all the people in our lives who aren't 100% supportive and positive. In-laws, bosses and honest accountants are facts of life. However, there are steps we can take to manage our responses to people, places and things that add stress. In the rest of this chapter, you'll find some great deep-breathing and anxiety-reducing techniques that will help you to stay focused on your goals for a happier you. You don't have to do everything – but you can choose to do something.

# Take a Deep Breath

If you could stop and take stock in the middle of a premenstrual meltdown, you'd probably notice that your breathing is rapid and shallow. When you're content and calm, your breaths become slow and deep. In her book, *Eight Weeks to Vibrant Health*, Dr. Hyla Cass counsels: "Think of a near miss in traffic. Your heart is pounding, your adrenaline pumping and your mind racing. If you

simply take 10 deep, slow breaths, these physiological symptoms related to stress will disappear in seconds and so will your anxiety."

She goes on to say, "Most of us breathe too shallowly. In fact, the lungs are the size of two footballs, and most of us are using only one-third of that capacity. Now is the time to develop the habit of breathing more deeply, so begin by spending a few short minutes every day doing just that."

## Dr. Cass' Deep-Breathing Exercise

Sit comfortably in a quiet place with your spine straight and relax your belly muscles.

As you inhale, let your abdomen expand. Feel your diaphragm being pulled down as your lungs fill with air from the bottom to the top. Pause briefly when you've inhaled fully.

As you exhale, gently contract your belly and squeeze the air out from top to bottom.

Repeat at your own pace.

You can do this in a few minutes any time you're feeling stressed and overwhelmed. It's a great way to calm yourself and recharge your batteries.

## Accentuate the Positive

It's time to pick up the pom-poms and become your own cheerleader. Many of us have a nasty habit of beating ourselves up almost constantly. We do it so often, we're not even aware of it.

Monitor your thoughts for a few days during PMS. Besides, "I wish there was more frosting on my cake," you're likely to

hear: "I hate myself for feeling this way" or "Everyone else is better at this than I am" or "I'll never stick to an exercise plan." This "toxic talk" does nothing but create doubt and low self-esteem. Would you say these negative things to a friend? Of course not! The question is why do you say them to yourself?

## Ixnay on the Hearsay

Many of us carry destructive messages we heard as children from teachers, coaches, and sadly, even parents, into adulthood; others hear the echoes of abusive relationships. The truth is that when you pay attention to those things, you're continuing the cycle by mistreating yourself and adding greatly to your stress. You're as vulnerable and as valuable as everyone else and deserve the same encouragement you'd give others.

Recognize your own uniqueness and your strengths. Say nice things to yourself. Instead of "I look like Keith Richards in drag" try "I'm working on feeling better and that's progress!" Substitute "I do things differently in my own unique way" for "Martha Stewart is the devil!" "Exercise is against my religion" becomes "I'm not in the habit yet, but I did walk last week and I know I can do it again." In time, encouraging self-talk will become a routine and positive action will follow.

## Take Me Away!

There are few things in life as relaxing as a bath. Long hot bubble baths can turn you into a new woman. Add candles and relaxing music, and voila! you have a spa getaway in the privacy of your own home. As a bonus, if you have a family, the bathroom is one of the only places in the house where you can lock the door, post a "do-not-disturb" sign and not feel remotely guilty.

Hot baths, ranging from 96F to 105F, soothe nerves, calm and relax the body, with the added benefits of stimulating the immune system and increasing circulation. Backaches and cramps can be vanquished by 15 minutes in a warm to hot tub. Stress and tension headaches melt away with the aid of a cool washcloth over your eyes.

In the bath, arm yourself with an array of essential oils to soothe the PMS primadonna within. Lavender, chamomile, sandalwood and amber are soothing; eucalyptus, mint, grapefruit and rosemary are

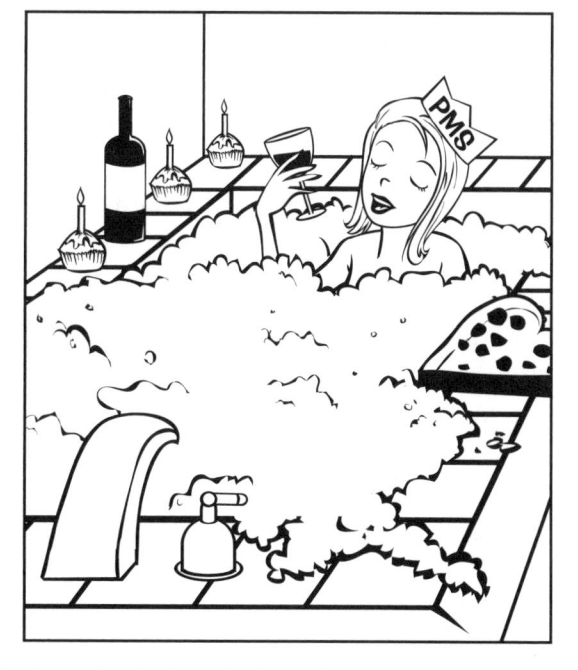

invigorating, while rose, geranium and bergamot can elevate your mood. You can find essential oils, which are much less expensive than pre-pared bath products, at most health or natural food stores. Sniff around a bit to find scents that tickle your nose and your fancy. Add a few drops to your bath and soak to your heart's and head's content.

Pass up extremely hot baths right before bed as they can make your heart race and keep you up. If your goal is to put yourself to sleep, a warm bath is a better choice. (Warning: Water temperatures above 101F put a strain on the heart as it works to dilate blood vessels in order to cool the body. If you suffer from heart disease, avoid these water temperatures.)

# Premenstrual Truce with a Masseuse

If you can stand being touched during **PMS**, massage promotes wellbeing and relaxation, and can make symptoms tolerable while you're making lifestyle adjustments. A good masseuse can drain the stress right out of you. There are many forms of massage that break down into two categories: relaxation and pain management. Most types of massage, from Swedish to deep tissue, sports to shiatsu, can be used for either. It's all about the degree of pressure being applied by your new best friend with the magic fingers. Be sure to tell your massage therapist what you have in mind and your goals.

Many forms of massage require you to be nude or in your underwear. Massage therapists take great pains to respect your privacy and will cover any part of you they're not working on with a warm towel or sheet. If you're not comfortable being in your birthday suit with a stranger, try one of the many massagers on the market, which focus on your head, neck, feet and hands. If cash-flow is a bigger problem than nudity, consider visiting a local massage school; therapists-in-training may be looking for "guinea pigs" and will offer their services at a reduced rate.

You can also use massage to connect with your significant other. There are therapeutic and erotic massage classes available in almost every town nationwide. They range from an evening to several weeks of touchy-feely fun and can do wonders for your stress level and your relationship. Your lover can learn to touch you in a way that is pleasing while you're premenstrual, and it's a special way to spend some time together.

# Choose Pleasure Over Pain

The next time one of your friends mutters "Somebody needs to get herself a little some-some" when faced with a cranky waitress, a bitchy bank teller or your PMS self, take it to heart. It's not exactly news that sex and the "Big O" have multiple benefits, but did you know that they can provide relief from PMS, tension and cramps?

Sex stimulates the immune system, warding off disease and like any exercise, it increases circulation providing relief from cramps. Sex with orgasm (clearly, the best kind) causes repeated contractions of the uterus and the body's musculature, relieving tightness and aiding in relaxation of the thighs, pelvis, glutes, back and all the other parts of a woman's body where she carries premenstrual tension.

A romp between the sheets can also increase your self-esteem, giving you a much needed premenstrual boost. During orgasm, our brains release endorphins, the body's natural opiates. Orgasm also promotes the release of oxytocin, a hormone that, in conjunction with estrogen, promotes a calming effect that no amount of chamomile tea can match. That calming effect may help us sleep, relieve migraines, and give us an overall feeling of wellbeing.

While sharing all this pleasure with a partner is a bonus, masturbation works just as well. There are countless studies on the positive benefits of sex and masturbation. Some recent scientific research even indicates that frequent sexual activity (with or without a partner) can increase your lifespan. So feel free to indulge yourself without guilt. It's all for a good cause.

# Stick it to PMS

The ancient Chinese art of acupuncture has won many converts in the U.S. A long tradition of treating menstrual problems with Traditional Chinese Medicine (see the section below) has proven it to be as effective as sweet and sour chicken is at treating a case of the munchies. (Or so we've been told.)

Your acupuncturist will develop a treatment plan that may include herbs and the use of very fine needles inserted into your skin to open blocked chi, or energy flow, through specific channels called meridians. The process is usually painless, not at all like what you experience when you accidentally prick your finger with a pin or a thorn. Most people report a slight numbing or tingling sensation when the needles are inserted, and a third-degree burning sensation when they breathe... We're just messin' with you on that last part.

## Crash Course: Traditional Chinese Medicine 101

James Tsai, L.Ac. and Andrew Wen, L.Ac.
Specialists in Traditional Chinese Medicine and Acupuncture

Although PMS is a western medical concept, Traditional Chinese Medicine (TCM) bases its diagnosis of PMS on the signs and symptoms of the individual. Through a time-honored method of data collection, a TCM practitioner formulates a single or multiple body organ diagnosis called a pattern. Once the pattern is established, a course of treatment can be tailored to a woman's needs. To understand the way that TCM practitioners work, here's some background on how they view the human body.

In TCM, Qi (pronounced "chee") is the essence of life, and yin and yang are the balance of life. Every bodily organ has its own Qi and its own balance, however, if an organ's Qi is in a state of blockage due to overwork, poor nutrition, family medical history or stress that alters the balance of yin and yang, then symptoms of PMS can occur.

TCM practitioners are trained to detect and interpret these often subtle signs and symptoms to formulate a diagnosis and treat the origin of the imbalance, just as the conductor of a symphony orchestra is trained to detect an instrument that is out of tune though an untrained ear may not hear the difference.

## Diagnostic Methods

When you visit a TCM practitioner, such as an acupuncturist, you can expect them to first inspect your eyes, tongue, hair, skin, body shape, etc. Next, auscultation involves listening to your breathing, coughing, sneezing, smelling your breath, etc. The practitioner will inquire about past and present family history, your energy level, your menstrual cycle, and so on. Finally, he or she will palpate, or feel, your pulse, chest and abdomen.

Based upon the pattern diagnosis, your TCM practitioner will develop a treatment principle. Acupuncture and herbs are the two main modalities used to balance your yin and yang and restore harmony with your other organs. Chinese herbal remedies with wonderful translations such as "True Warrior Decoction" and "Return the Spleen Pill" may be prescribed to supplement acupuncture treatment.

# PMS Prognosis

Every individual's genetic makeup and medical history varies. For example, a condition with a 10-year history will require more treatment than PMS with only a three-month history. However, as a general guideline with all menstrual problems, two or three visits a week for an average of three menstrual cycles is a common course of treatment. In most cases, patients will notice a reduction in the severity of PMS after only one month of treatment.

A typical licensed acupuncturist undergoes an average of 2,500 to 3,000 hours of training. To find a qualified acupuncturist in your area, log onto the website of the National Certification Commission for Acupuncture and Oriental Medicine at www.nccaom.org.

# Other TCM Options for PMS

Qi Gong (Chinese energy exercise therapy) can be very effective when practiced regularly. Try the following exercise:

Lie down comfortably on a flat surface and close your eyes. Breathe evenly and place the tip of the tongue gently against the roof of your mouth toward the upper teeth. Using your navel as the center of a circle, place your left hand over your right hand. Move your hands slowly in a clockwise direction, 36 times, and count silently while thinking, "I feel relaxed and healthy." Repeat in a counterclockwise direction.

At the end of the exercise, place your hands three inches below your navel. Spend several minutes paying attention to how relaxed your body feels. This exercise should be done 2 to 3 times daily for 10 days before your period and continued until it's over.

# Tai Chi for PMS

This ancient art of moving meditation dates back hundreds of years, and is practiced by more than a billion people. Tai Chi is a method of self-defense, relaxation and healing that consists of gentle and fluid motions suitable for all ages.

Practicing Tai Chi on a regular basis can decrease stress, increase energy, prevent illness, improve concentration, strengthen the mind and body, and slow the effects of aging. Check with your local gym, YWCA, or look for a Tai Chi video for at-home use.

# Under Pressure

If the idea of needles is more frightening to you than PMS, consider acupressure. It uses the same basic principles as acupuncture without the needles, instead applying pressure to key points on the body to stimulate your natural self-healing abilities. The therapeutic touch of acupressure reduces tension, increases circulation and can promote deep relaxation.

If you do a little research on acupressure, you'll find there are 365 points, each one aptly named. These names offer insight into either a point's benefits or location. For instance, the name "Hidden Clarity" refers to the mental benefit of the point: It clears the mind. The "Three Mile Point" gives you an energy boost and is used by runners to increase stamina and endurance.

Unlike acupuncture, you can try acupressure at home. You can perform the exercises yourself, or ask a friend or loved one to help. Following are some acupressure exercises that you can use anytime.

Try to do them somewhere warm and quiet. Hold each point indicated in the exercise with a steady pressure for one to three minutes, using the tips or balls of the fingers. The acupressure point may feel tender indicating that the energy pathway, or meridian, is blocked. During treatment, the tenderness should slowly go away.

✳ **For Back Pain:**

Lie on your back on a comfortable surface, such as a rug or mat, with your knees bent and your feet flat on the floor. Make two fists. Place your fists, knuckles up, under your back just above your waistline and about an inch from either side of your spine. Let your knuckles settle into your muscles and apply sustained gentle pressure. Breathe deeply, counting to five as you inhale and to five as you exhale. Do this exercise for three minutes.

✳ **For Headaches:**

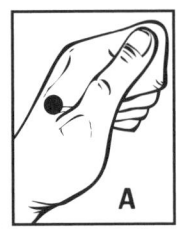

This is a great exercise to do anywhere: at home, at the office, or during dinner with the in-laws. Using the thumb and forefinger of your right hand, pinch the muscle mass below and between your left thumb and forefinger (see diagram A).

Pinch this point as hard as you can, applying deep pressure for 15 to 30 seconds. The point may be very tender. Repeat on the right hand.

✳ **For Stress:**

The Four Gates is a traditional Chinese point combination that has been used for centuries. You'll need someone to assist you. Work first on one side of the body and then on the other. Ask your helper to apply pressure simultaneously to the points in diagrams A (above) & B (on the opposite page). Hold for 30 seconds, applying light pressure. Then, repeat on the other side.

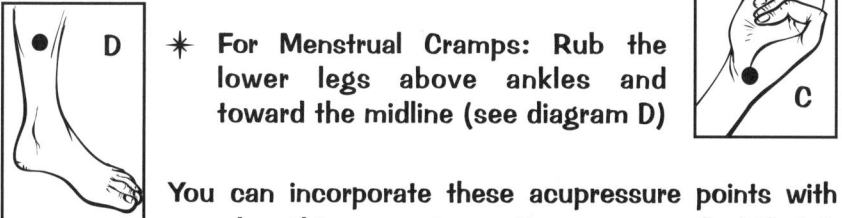

If you don't have an acupressure buddy, try the following points by yourself. For each, massage, applying light pressure with your thumb or forefinger for 30 seconds, then release. Repeat two to three times throughout the day.

✳ For Irritability (also part of the Four Gates technique): Massage the top of feet in between the large and second toes (see diagram B)

✳ For Anxiety: Apply pressure to the inner wrist (see diagram C)

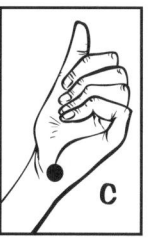

✳ For Menstrual Cramps: Rub the lower legs above ankles and toward the midline (see diagram D)

You can incorporate these acupressure points with your breathing exercises. Some women find that it helps to visualize themselves as healthy and PMS-free while applying pressure to the points. If acupressure is new to you or a bit confusing, visit a professional. Many massage therapists are also trained in acupressure, or can refer you to an acupressure specialist. Remember, this is supposed to relieve your stress, not add to it.

## "Om" at Home

Meditation, like spiritual belief, can take many forms and have a calming effect on mind and body. When practiced regularly, prayer or meditation can clear away mental clutter, soothe physical pain and provide the quiet strength to persevere in the face of PMS and other stressors.

Meditation can be as simple as sitting in contemplation. Many types of meditation suggest that you focus on something, such as a word or phrase, known as a mantra. You'll need a quiet place with as little stimulation as possible and you may have to try several times before finding the right mantra or focus for you. One of the keys to success is not to worry about whether you're doing it right or criticize yourself for doing it wrong. (Falling asleep while meditating is common for beginners and just means that you need a little shut-eye.)

Some women find it easier to take a class or use self-hypnosis or relaxation CDs that are targeted to a particular goal (weight loss, smoking cessation, mastering anger or anxiety, etc.). The audio will guide you through breathing exercises, creative visualization and other techniques to help you achieve your objective. Whatever you decide to try, meditation, self-hypnosis or prayer, do it as often as possible. It's a time for you to focus on yourself and your healing.

## "Letting Go" Exercise

Sit comfortably in a quiet room. Close your eyes. Listen to the rhythm of your breathing. Imagine that you are in a warm, wonderful place like a flower-filled meadow or on top of a mountain with the sun and a gentle breeze caressing you.

Choose a word that inspires you, such as "healing" or "peace" or a phrase such as "I am healthy and strong." Try "om" the original mantra, an ancient word believed to be the boat that helps one to cross the rivers of fear. You can even select nonsense words just because you like the way they sound, such as "splish splash" or "whoosh." Many people find that two syllable words work well; inhale on the first syllable and exhale on the second.

Relax the muscles throughout your body, from your toes to the top of your head. Don't forget about your stomach, buttocks, chest, shoulders and facial muscles where women often carry stress. As you repeat your word or phrase silently, exhale the stress from your body. Feel your body softening and melting into the chair.

If unwanted thoughts pop into your head, just acknowledge them and send them away. Keep breathing and focusing on your mantra for 10 to 20 minutes (start with a few minutes and work your way up) then open your eyes. Resume your day, refreshed and renewed.

# Laughter Is the Best Medicine

PMS is not often a laughing matter, especially when it feels like you're uterus-deep in emotional quicksand. However, once all males are out of the room, most women would be hard-pressed not to find a little bit of humor in their often unpredictable predicament.

Scientists have begun to study the correlation between health and humor. They've added a laugh-o-meter to their array of instruments and discovered that adults laugh approximately 15 times per day, while children chuckle more than 400 times a day. Somehow, between childhood and adulthood, playground and parenthood, grown-ups lose a few hundred laughs a day. By learning to smile and laugh again, more easily and more often, we can make profound and positive changes to our health and welfare.

The immune system is stimulated by laughter. Laughter acts as the body's safety valve countering stress. When we release tension by laughing, for example, listening to Kathy Griffin do her stand-up or a divorce attorney trying to sound sincere, the

elevated levels of the body's stress hormones drop back to normal. Researchers have also found that laughter causes the tissue that forms the inner lining of the blood vessels to dilate, increasing blood flow in the same way as aerobic exercise, minus the workout wedgies. As the vessels relax and expand, more oxygen is carried in the blood to your heart and brain.

If nothing about your situation seems funny, consider Laughter Yoga. In 1995, a physician from India developed the practice, which combines simulated laughter and gentle yoga breathing that miraculously turns into real belly laughter when practiced as a group.

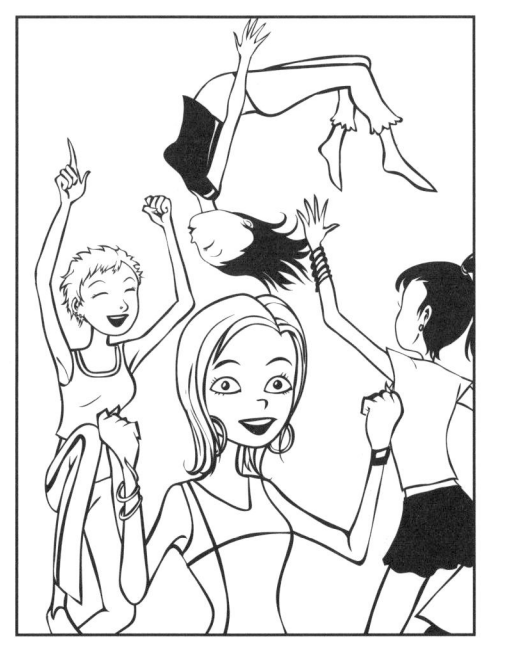

If you want to skip the yoga but still need a chuckle, check out a laughter club. Leaders guide members through a series of funny moves – anything from imitating penguins to pretending to walk over hot sand – to trigger laughter. Worldwide, there are about 3,500 laughter clubs that have helped countless people discover the mental and physical health benefits of a good giggle. The therapeutic advantages have convinced corporations, nursing homes, schools and the Cancer Treatment Centers of America® to show patients and their families how to make laughter an important part of their curriculum. If laughter is contagious, it's one "ailment" you won't mind catching.

## An Optimistic Outlook

Try changing your perspective, and consider the upside of PMS.

* Your significant other is suddenly agreeing with everything you say.
* Merely pointing to a calendar stops anyone from questioning the raw cookie dough on your nightstand.
* You can earn big bucks for demolition.
* Telemarketers won't be calling again anytime soon.
* Alone time is a given.
* You don't have to invent an excuse to avoid sex — no one's asking!

## Break "The Curse"

When you're under pressure, chances are that the person who gets the short end of the stick is you. If that weren't the case, you'd have addressed your PMS long ago. The great news is that you're doing it now and by conquering your PMS, you'll be in much better physical and emotional shape to tackle the important things while still tending to yourself.

No matter what you choose to do, whether it's deep-breathing, positive self-talk, baths, massage, acupuncture, a laughter club or all of the above, it's important that you do something for yourself. Take good care of your mind and body. Applaud your successes and remember that there are no failures, just temporary setbacks that are opportunities for learning and progress and even laughter! You may not be a superwoman but, day by day, you're moving closer to becoming a PMS-free one.

# A Note From Our Relationship Coaches

These days, most of us are focused on growth and improvement. You spend precious time and countless dollars improving your diet, exercise patterns, attitude, state of mind, etc., and yet, you haven't achieved mastery of your PMS. As tough as it is for you, contemplate what it might be like for your main squeeze to live in the ever-present shadow of the "Big P."

In the following chapters, you'll find some valuable coaching on how to tame the monster within while protecting loved ones during your most trying premenstrual times. Learn to identify and manage your emotions and response in "The 'I' of the Storm" and discover how to communicate positively with each other – PMS or not – in "Getting Well, Together." These coaching tips will provide access to some much needed understanding and compassion for yourself and others.

With a little encouragement, you can restore harmony to your life and relationship. Read on and you'll discover how to love yourself – and your loved ones – back to premenstrual health.

—Elizabeth Goodman & Herb Tanzer

# The "I" of the Storm

PMS can feel like a Category 5 storm that's bearing down on your emotional wellbeing. The upset, anger and anxiety are the rain, wind and swirling debris, and like a natural disaster, they can lay waste to your sense of self and your environment. But, at the center of the storm – the "I" of the PMS storm – is a calm and quiet place. Navigating through the danger zone to that place may be difficult, but it is possible.

## Stop the Madness!

When everything feels out of control and the emotional storm is about to make landfall, there is one powerful move and that is to… STOP! Stop and pay attention to the automatic thinking that has taken over your mind and body. We all have ongoing streams of negative thinking and automatic reactions, which may be intensified during the PMS hurricane. Those automatic reactions echo your personal history and past upsets, and usually have nothing to do with the present situation.

Here's an example: Let's say your significant other innocently asks after dinner, "Would you like to go to for a walk?" His words trigger a lightning-fast conversation in your head about what those words mean and why they irritate you. That conversation might sound something like:

"Walk? Is he insane? I've been working all day, I'm exhausted and everything hurts. He must think I'm fat. That's why he wants me to go for a walk. What's the use? He's probably planning to leave me for some pencil-thin bimbo!"

And on and on it goes. Before you know it, you've overreacted and all but blown the house down. It happened so fast you probably didn't even notice: In the midst of the upset, you just made up a whole story, which triggered your ancient insecurities and fundamental feelings of unworthiness. These old companions, in turn, further intensify the storm.

This automatic response is part of being human. However, if you are conscious of the automatic behavior operating here, then this moment occurs as a place to **STOP** and regain your power and control. Suspending the automatic reaction returns you to a less emotionally charged starting place and allows you to intelligently evaluate if there's any actual upset in what the poor guy said.

# What's So

When you **STOP** and note your automatic thinking, you'll have a chance to separate the facts from your fiction about them. This will give you the "What's So" to work with. Think of it as truth that's free of hormones and history.

**The path to "What's So":**

* **What interpretations have you made?** ...he thinks I'm fat!
* **What emotions have arisen automatically?**...insecurity, fear
* **What decisions have you made about people, things or situations?** ...I've decided his friendly suggestion to walk together means something sinister
* **What have you demanded or are about to demand?** ...that he go play in traffic
* **What happened versus your interpretation of it?** ...umm, I think he wanted to go for a walk together and I was about to call Weight Watchers® or a divorce lawyer!

Separating what happened from your *interpretation* of what happened leaves you in a place called "What's So." Before you call your girlfriends to tell them that the bastard is leaving you, consider the hormonal hurricane that may have temporarily wiped out your ability to assess reality, or "What's So." You owe it to yourself and your baffled partner to consider the facts before you react.

## So What?

Finding your way to the facts means separating the stories you have attached to those facts. For example, THE STORY might be that you are worried about your relationship: you might feel lousy and insecure because PMS has helped you pack on a few pounds, or maybe you're lugging around an idea that you're not the ideal woman.

THE FACTS are your husband is with you and he wants to go for a walk! Seeing the naked "What's So" (just the facts, ma'am) devoid of interpretation, removes all the significance your story has added to the facts. At this point, the troubling theatrics can be replaced with a refreshing "So What?" – a very powerful place from which to act.

## Now What?

The question after all the drama is over is simply: "Now what?" If you're tired of being tossed around by all that distress you're helping to create, it's time to rewrite the stories you tell yourself, so you can move past your inappropriate reactions. That is the way into the calm, still, place at the center of the PMS storm.

"Now What?" is the time to work on changing your perspective. Can you wipe all story slates clean, and begin from a place where the people in your lives don't have hidden agendas, ulterior motives or any power that you don't give them? Whether it's your boss who's afraid of losing her job and snaps at you, or your mechanic who's just giving you his professional opinion when he says your brakes are shot, sometimes surface value is all there is. Why attach anything else to it? When you drop the story, or negative internal dialogue, and stick with the "What's So," you'll begin to really listen to what people are saying and stop reacting automatically. Giving up the righteousness of your story allows you to move forward to a healthier – and more peaceful – quality of life.

## What's What

Whenever you're confronted by a problem that seems unsolvable or a situation you'd like to change, like PMS, you can use this approach. Remember:

✳ STOP! Notice your automatic thinking.

✳ What meaning have you attached? What story have you told yourself?

✳ Figure out the facts, the "What's So" at the center of the mess.

✳ Once you have the facts without the story you added, you have replaced the significance with a big fat, juicy "So what?"

✳ From the "So what?" you go directly to "Now what?" and choose what actions are appropriate.

It may take time for you to notice your automatic thinking, and even more time for you to let go of your learned reactions. But, when you gain mastery over the chatter in your head and say goodbye to all the turmoil, you'll find the calm in the storm. With a little practice, that calm can be you.

*Honi, the Circlemaker, traveled from town to town. In each new place, he would find a stick and carefully inscribe a circle around himself. Though he traveled far and wide, no matter where Honi was, he was always in the center.*

—from a Talmudic proverb

# Getting Well, Together

Since the first man (or woman) constructed a myth to explain the rising sun, humankind has done its best to cope with the mysteries of the world. Not much has changed. When the ups and downs of life are difficult to fathom, we try to make sense of them by creating modern day fables to explain our troubles. These tall tales often sound a lot like finger pointing.

Women faced with PMS run through a laundry list of suspects in their reproductive years: clueless parents, helter-skelter hormones, bad genes, imperfect boyfriends, insensitive gynecologists, demanding bosses, or even God for cursing them with womanhood. Men are just as likely to go hunting for a PMS culprit, but to what end? Brain researchers have found that when people are scared, hurt or angry (all unpleasant side effects of dealing with PMS) they're physiologically incapable of thinking straight.

Man or woman, it's easier to assign blame than to fix problems. However, blame equals powerlessness. When you blame an outside force, a boss or an inescapable fact of life like hormones, you render yourself powerless. How can you manage or change something that's not your fault? The one constant in life's series of unrelated occurrences is you. You are always at the center of the circle. What if no one is to blame for your PMS but someone is responsible? What if the responsible person is you?

# Acceptance

PMS is a fact of life. It is real and it is mediated by hormones. You may not be able to choose whether you have PMS, but you can choose who you want to be with PMS while you treat it. Think about it this way: If you had to create a fictional email address for yourself during your worst premenstrual days, would it be jane@ravinglunatic.com or jane@peacemaker.com?

You can dramatize your PMS with Oscar®-worthy meltdowns, or practice acceptance or "non-interference." Instead of resisting PMS through denial or blame – and remember that what you resist persists – you can acknowledge and take responsibility for it by gaining altitude and perspective. Imagine that you are soaring high above yourself and that you are able to put emotional distance between you and your PMS. This altitude gives you freedom to choose how you're going to respond to the hormonal bombardment.

# Red Flag Alert

Have you ever tripped on uneven pavement or an unexpected stair? Those signs cautioning you to "Watch Your Step" are there for a reason. Imagine your significant other or your coworkers, blindly walking along, unaware that there's an obstacle in their path – you with PMS. Ignoring or denying your PMS is equivalent to skipping through a minefield with your loved ones in tow. Chances are everyone's going to get blown up.

You can exercise responsibility for your genetic and hormonal makeup without dramatizing it by communicating openly. It can be as simple as saying: "My hormones are raging and I apologize upfront" or "I'm a little emotional today." If you're talking with a

loved one, invite them to share responsibility by adding, "What I need from you is to be sensitive to the fact that I'm a little crazy right now and I would like you to sit with me, hug me, etc."

# Off the Right Track

You can make a choice to be happy. We all know someone who is passionate about being right. He's the one who'll stick to his guns no matter what logic he's confronted with; she's the one who'll argue 'til she's blue in the face to prove her point, no matter how many people she alienates in the process. These people are seldom well-liked, and in spite of "being right," they're usually not happy. Your life proves what you are committed to. Are you committed to being right or being happy?

Most couples have the same fight over and over again. It may assume different forms, but it's ultimately about each person's "rightness," whether it's the best route to the mall or whose turn it is to do household chores. Over time, we tend to get "dug in" or stuck. We're sure that we don't like X, don't want to try Y, can't change Z. By focusing all our attention on a particular point of view, we close ourselves off to change. As comedienne Lily Tomlin famously said, "The mind is like a parachute. It only works when it's open!"

If your partner is convinced that PMS is all in your mind, he's not going to accept that a massage and a little compassion could change your family politics for the better. Similarly, if you're committed to being stuck with PMS, you're unlikely to investigate supplements or lifestyle changes. Why? You're more attached to being right about your PMS than being happy. Allowing that there are alternative ways to think about PMS, and life's other challenges, opens a world of possibilities and hope.

# Choose What You Think, Think What You Choose

Humans are highly suggestible creatures. If someone says "don't think about pink elephants," you can't help but conjure up images of bubblegum-pink pachyderms. Think of yourself as a victim of your hormonal fluctuations and you'll drag through your PMS days each month, downtrodden and hopeless. If, on the other hand, you decide – and it's a conscious choice – to view those days as an opportunity to reach for the brass ring of health and happiness, you might still be crampy but your focus will be on healing. Simply put, where your attention goes, your energy flows.

Winning the war with PMS is like playing poker. You have no choice in the cards you're dealt, just in how you play them. While you can't change biology or genetics, *who you are*, you can change *how you are* by altering how you think. The truth is that what you experience doesn't determine what you feel; instead, what you *think* and *say* about those experiences determines how you feel.

When you're upset, what are the thoughts associated with your feelings? If your spouse forgets an item on the grocery list, is there a broken record of "He never does X... He always says Y" running endlessly in your head? If someone cuts you off in traffic, do you scream obscenities? Do these thoughts and words calm you down or get you more worked up? Is your energy flowing to positive or negative thoughts and feelings? If the answer is that you're focused on the negative, what alternative thoughts might make you feel good?

Consider your surroundings. You enjoy greater freedoms than any known throughout history. You have food and shelter, and the leisure time to read a good book. You are loved and you have friends. There are countless blessings on which you can focus your attention. Or, you can keep thinking negative thoughts and see where they take you.

How you view your circumstances applies not only to PMS, but also to the broader context of life. Go to work thinking "I have to be here" instead of "I am lucky that I get to be here" and your days will seem endless. Sit down for a heart-to-heart with a loved one with a bad attitude and the outcome will be the same – bad. If a couple's attention is consistently focused on arguments and discord (fueled by their "rightness") then their energy can't be directed to healthy communication. You can use PMS to start a dialogue with your significant other that's positive, ultimately leading to empowerment and happiness.

# Relate & Communicate

Neuroscientists at the Universities of Wisconsin and Virginia recently completed a study on a husband's touch. The results showed that women under extreme stress felt immediate relief at the touch of their husbands' hands. This isn't news.

Says Elizabeth, "When I had PMS, there was an inordinate amount of energy coursing through my body. I was very scattered and less able to function effectively. Being touched or hugged took all the scattered energy and focused it, grounding me."

The energy that Elizabeth's talking about is like lightning: lethal if it hits you head on. Being hugged focused her tension so it

could dissipate; being touched released that negative energy, alleviating some of her symptoms. Scientists don't yet know all the reasons why, but they do know that physical contact makes us feel secure and calm.

Of course, the last thing your significant other wants to do is to get close to the source of turmoil; even the most primitive organisms automatically move away from a disturbance. Faced with a woman who's in the midst of raging PMS, men know instinctually to get away from the source of the aggravation. They are more likely to think, "I know what to do...book a flight to Mongolia!" than "she could use a hug right about now."

It takes every ounce of self-control and discipline to move in the direction of the upset, but the only way out for both of you is to get connected, whether by touch or a kind word. It's your responsibility to tell the people who love you that you need that contact so they can start helping and stop being wrong all the time.

# The Race to Sanity

Throughout this book, we've emphasized that PMS is a biological condition and women who experience its monthly upsets aren't insane. However, when everything around us is spiraling out of control, life can feel a little looney.

As you work on your relationships and communication, here's a good rule of thumb to remember: Whoever gets "sane" (or well) first takes care of the other one. In all likelihood, while you're still battling PMS, your guy is going to be first to limp across the

finish line.   As you begin your 100th disagreement about something minor, rather than engaging, keep in mind that this is a volatile time and before you know it, a spat can turn into a marital meltdown.   Disengage. If you're arguing over where to park or what to have for dinner, give in!   It's a great way to restore a little peace and harmony and what did it really cost you?

It comes back to the notion of whether it's more important to you to be right or to be happy.   We're betting on happy.

# Monthly "Monstrual" Chart

Keeping track of your periods and your premenstrual symptoms are important tools in the fight against **PMS**. You may know that you feel like something the cat dragged in before your period, but until you have a record of your actual symptoms and evidence that they recur reliably prior to menstruation, it will be tough to treat them.

In the following pages, you'll find two sample charts and six blank ones for you to fill in. In the samples for January and February, you'll notice that our Premenstrual Princess gets her period every 28 days. She also has anxiety, back pain, bloating and food binges in the days leading up to her period. She may have thought that her headaches were another symptom of PMS, but the chart indicates that she has them throughout the month at irregular intervals. That's a good indication that PMS isn't to blame for her throbbing head at all.

Use the six blank Monthly "Monstrual" Charts to find your own premenstrual pattern. Fill in the month, the days that you have your period, and most importantly, your PMS symptoms and when they occur, and you'll be well on your way to premenstrual freedom.

## JANUARY

| | Menstruation | Anxiety | Headaches | Back Pain | Bloating | Other |
|---|---|---|---|---|---|---|
| 1 | | X | | | | |
| 2 | | X | | | | |
| 3 | | X | | | X | |
| 4 | | X | | | X | |
| 5 | | X | | | X | |
| 6 | | X | X | X | X | |
| 7 | | X | | X | X | |
| 8 | | X | | X | X | food binges |
| 9 | | X | | X | X | food binges |
| 10 | ☹ | | | X | X | irritability |
| 11 | ☹ | | | X | | cramps |
| 12 | ☹ | | | | | |
| 13 | ☹ | | | | | |
| 14 | ☹ | | | | | |
| 15 | | | | | | |
| 16 | | | | | | |
| 17 | | | | | | |
| 18 | | | X | | | |
| 19 | | | X | | | |
| 20 | | | | | | |
| 21 | | | | | | |
| 22 | | | | | | |
| 23 | | | | | | |
| 24 | | | | | | |
| 25 | | | X | | | |
| 26 | | | | | | |
| 27 | | | X | | | |
| 28 | | | | | | |
| 29 | | | | | | |
| 30 | | X | | | | |
| 31 | | X | | | | |

# FEBRUARY

| | Menstruation | Anxiety | Headaches | Back Pain | Bloating | Other |
|---|---|---|---|---|---|---|
| 1 | | X | | | | |
| 2 | | X | | | X | |
| 3 | | X | | | X | |
| 4 | | X | | | X | |
| 5 | | X | | | X | |
| 6 | | X | X | | X | |
| 7 | | X | | X | X | food binges |
| 8 | | X | | X | X | food binges |
| 9 | | X | | X | X | food binges |
| 10 | | X | | X | X | food binges |
| 11 | ☹ | | | X | | acne/cramps |
| 12 | ☹ | | | | | |
| 13 | ☹ | | | | | |
| 14 | ☹ | | X | | | cramps |
| 15 | ☹ | | | | | |
| 16 | | | | | | |
| 17 | | | | | | |
| 18 | | | | | | |
| 19 | | | | | | |
| 20 | | | | | | irritability |
| 21 | | | X | | | |
| 22 | | | X | | | |
| 23 | | | X | | | |
| 24 | | | | | | |
| 25 | | | | | | |
| 26 | | | | | | |
| 27 | | | | | | |
| 28 | | | | | | |
| 29 | | | | | | |
| 30 | | | | | | |
| 31 | | | | | | |

# The Princess and the PMS

**Month:**

| | Menstruation | | | | Other |
|---|---|---|---|---|---|
| 1 | | | | | |
| 2 | | | | | |
| 3 | | | | | |
| 4 | | | | | |
| 5 | | | | | |
| 6 | | | | | |
| 7 | | | | | |
| 8 | | | | | |
| 9 | | | | | |
| 10 | | | | | |
| 11 | | | | | |
| 12 | | | | | |
| 13 | | | | | |
| 14 | | | | | |
| 15 | | | | | |
| 16 | | | | | |
| 17 | | | | | |
| 18 | | | | | |
| 19 | | | | | |
| 20 | | | | | |
| 21 | | | | | |
| 22 | | | | | |
| 23 | | | | | |
| 24 | | | | | |
| 25 | | | | | |
| 26 | | | | | |
| 27 | | | | | |
| 28 | | | | | |
| 29 | | | | | |
| 30 | | | | | |
| 31 | | | | | |

Monthly "Menstrual" Chart

**Month:**

| | Menstruation | | | | | Other |
|---|---|---|---|---|---|---|
| 1 | | | | | | |
| 2 | | | | | | |
| 3 | | | | | | |
| 4 | | | | | | |
| 5 | | | | | | |
| 6 | | | | | | |
| 7 | | | | | | |
| 8 | | | | | | |
| 9 | | | | | | |
| 10 | | | | | | |
| 11 | | | | | | |
| 12 | | | | | | |
| 13 | | | | | | |
| 14 | | | | | | |
| 15 | | | | | | |
| 16 | | | | | | |
| 17 | | | | | | |
| 18 | | | | | | |
| 19 | | | | | | |
| 20 | | | | | | |
| 21 | | | | | | |
| 22 | | | | | | |
| 23 | | | | | | |
| 24 | | | | | | |
| 25 | | | | | | |
| 26 | | | | | | |
| 27 | | | | | | |
| 28 | | | | | | |
| 29 | | | | | | |
| 30 | | | | | | |
| 31 | | | | | | |

**Month:**

| | Menstruation | | | | | Other |
|---|---|---|---|---|---|---|
| 1 | | | | | | |
| 2 | | | | | | |
| 3 | | | | | | |
| 4 | | | | | | |
| 5 | | | | | | |
| 6 | | | | | | |
| 7 | | | | | | |
| 8 | | | | | | |
| 9 | | | | | | |
| 10 | | | | | | |
| 11 | | | | | | |
| 12 | | | | | | |
| 13 | | | | | | |
| 14 | | | | | | |
| 15 | | | | | | |
| 16 | | | | | | |
| 17 | | | | | | |
| 18 | | | | | | |
| 19 | | | | | | |
| 20 | | | | | | |
| 21 | | | | | | |
| 22 | | | | | | |
| 23 | | | | | | |
| 24 | | | | | | |
| 25 | | | | | | |
| 26 | | | | | | |
| 27 | | | | | | |
| 28 | | | | | | |
| 29 | | | | | | |
| 30 | | | | | | |
| 31 | | | | | | |

# Monthly "Monstrual" Chart

**Month:**

| | Menstruation | | | | | Other |
|---|---|---|---|---|---|---|
| 1 | | | | | | |
| 2 | | | | | | |
| 3 | | | | | | |
| 4 | | | | | | |
| 5 | | | | | | |
| 6 | | | | | | |
| 7 | | | | | | |
| 8 | | | | | | |
| 9 | | | | | | |
| 10 | | | | | | |
| 11 | | | | | | |
| 12 | | | | | | |
| 13 | | | | | | |
| 14 | | | | | | |
| 15 | | | | | | |
| 16 | | | | | | |
| 17 | | | | | | |
| 18 | | | | | | |
| 19 | | | | | | |
| 20 | | | | | | |
| 21 | | | | | | |
| 22 | | | | | | |
| 23 | | | | | | |
| 24 | | | | | | |
| 25 | | | | | | |
| 26 | | | | | | |
| 27 | | | | | | |
| 28 | | | | | | |
| 29 | | | | | | |
| 30 | | | | | | |
| 31 | | | | | | |

**The Princess and the PMS**

**Month:**

| | Menstruation | | | | | Other |
|---|---|---|---|---|---|---|
| 1 | | | | | | |
| 2 | | | | | | |
| 3 | | | | | | |
| 4 | | | | | | |
| 5 | | | | | | |
| 6 | | | | | | |
| 7 | | | | | | |
| 8 | | | | | | |
| 9 | | | | | | |
| 10 | | | | | | |
| 11 | | | | | | |
| 12 | | | | | | |
| 13 | | | | | | |
| 14 | | | | | | |
| 15 | | | | | | |
| 16 | | | | | | |
| 17 | | | | | | |
| 18 | | | | | | |
| 19 | | | | | | |
| 20 | | | | | | |
| 21 | | | | | | |
| 22 | | | | | | |
| 23 | | | | | | |
| 24 | | | | | | |
| 25 | | | | | | |
| 26 | | | | | | |
| 27 | | | | | | |
| 28 | | | | | | |
| 29 | | | | | | |
| 30 | | | | | | |
| 31 | | | | | | |

# Monthly "Menstrual" Chart

**Month:**

| | Menstruation | | | | Other |
|---|---|---|---|---|---|
| 1 | | | | | |
| 2 | | | | | |
| 3 | | | | | |
| 4 | | | | | |
| 5 | | | | | |
| 6 | | | | | |
| 7 | | | | | |
| 8 | | | | | |
| 9 | | | | | |
| 10 | | | | | |
| 11 | | | | | |
| 12 | | | | | |
| 13 | | | | | |
| 14 | | | | | |
| 15 | | | | | |
| 16 | | | | | |
| 17 | | | | | |
| 18 | | | | | |
| 19 | | | | | |
| 20 | | | | | |
| 21 | | | | | |
| 22 | | | | | |
| 23 | | | | | |
| 24 | | | | | |
| 25 | | | | | |
| 26 | | | | | |
| 27 | | | | | |
| 28 | | | | | |
| 29 | | | | | |
| 30 | | | | | |
| 31 | | | | | |

# Remedy Chart

In "It's a Balancing Act: PMS & Supplements," you read about the role vitamins, minerals, amino acids and herbal remedies can play in reducing or eliminating your PMS symptoms. On the following pages, we've included a reference of supplements, their uses and possible precautions.

When shopping for supplements and herbs, be sure to buy from reputable sources. Look for supplements labeled "free of sugars, salt, artificial colors, preservatives and lactose." If you're buying a multi-vitamin, be sure it contains the major vitamins and minerals in amounts close to the recommended daily intake guidelines. You'll probably need to buy a calcium and magnesium supplement separately; a pill packed with other nutrients can't hold enough calcium or magnesium to make a dent in your PMS.

Look for herbal remedies that are standardized. In standardized herbs, one primary ingredient is the marker or most active ingredient; for example, in Feverfew, the marker is parthenolides. Standardizing ensures that you get the same amount of the active ingredient from brand to brand or batch to batch. While you're at it, check the expiration date; extracts, tinctures and tablets all have a limited shelf-life. If you want to avoid animal by-products, look for "gelatin-free" on capsule labels.

Please consult your healthcare practitioner before adding any supplements to your diet. Remember that there's no one-size-fits-all solution to PMS. You may need to experiment with supplements and herbs to find the combination that works best for you.

# The Princess and the PMS

| Remedy | Symptoms | Precautions |
|---|---|---|
| B Vitamins | fatigue anxiety stress | excessive doses of B6 can cause neurological problems |
| Black Cohosh | symptoms of peri-menopause | none known |
| Calcium | pain depression food cravings stress/anxiety | none at recommended dose |
| Chasteberry | mood swings hot flashes relieves heavy/ irregular periods breast pain headaches anger | do not use with hormone therapy or anti-depressants; do not take if pregnant; rare reports of headaches, weight gain, nausea |
| Damiana | low libido | none known |
| Dong Quai | symptoms of hormonal imbalance | do not use during period as it intensifies bleeding |
| Essential Fatty Acids: Omega 3 and 6 | depression inflammation and joint pain | do not take with blood-thinning medication |

Remedy Chart

| Remedy | Symptoms | Precautions |
|---|---|---|
| L-Tyrosine | anxiety<br>tension<br>insomnia<br>depression<br>fatigue | do not take with MAO inhibitors, or if you have high blood pressure, melanoma, if pregnant or nursing; works best taken with vitamin B6 |
| L-Tryptophan | anxiety<br>tension<br>insomnia<br>depression<br>carbohydrate cravings | do not take with anti-depressants; may cause dizziness, drowsiness, dry mouth |
| GABA<br>(Gamma Aminobutyric Acid) | anxiety<br>tension<br>insomnia<br>depression | high doses may cause nausea and vomiting |
| Feverfew | headaches<br>migraines | do not take with anti-coagulant drugs; do not take when pregnant |
| Evening Primrose Oil | breast tenderness<br>depression<br>irritability<br>water retention | may cause stomach upset, headache, rash |

| Remedy | Symptoms | Precautions |
|--------|----------|-------------|
| Magnesium | muscle spasms constipation anxiety water retention headaches | none at recommended dose; higher amounts may have a laxative effect; get the chelated form |
| Red Clover | perimenopause low estrogen | none known |
| St. John's Wort | depression anxiety | may cause allergic reaction, rash, stomach upset; do not use if pregnant or nursing |
| Tango | low libido lack of energy | do not take if pregnant or nursing |
| Valerian Root | anxiety tension insomnia | will increase the effect of other sedatives, including muscle relaxants and antihistamines; avoid alcohol and narcotics |

Information regarding uses and precautions are for guidance only, and you should discuss all use of vitamins, minerals, herbs and other supplements with your physician. See "Our Lawyers Made Us Say This..." at the beginning of this book.

# About the Authors

## Elizabeth Goodman

For most of her life, Elizabeth Goodman has applied her heart's passion for helping men and women bridge the gender gap by empowering them to communicate more effectively and compassionately. Through her successful career in personal coaching, she leads couples to understand how PMS can affect their relationships and how they can work together to nurture, strengthen and preserve those bonds.

In concert with her commitment to inspire truthful communication and intimacy, she is the co-author of *The Owner's Manual: The Essential Guide to the One You Love*, a book designed to reveal direct insights into what's really important to your beloved. Born in Philadelphia, Ms. Goodman is a former political consultant and fundraiser. She currently lives with her husband and partner, Herb Tanzer, in North San Diego County. Contact her at Elizabeth@PMSCentral.com.

## Neal Barnard, M.D.

Clinical researcher and author Neal Barnard, M.D., is a leading advocate for health, nutrition and higher standards in research. He is president of the Physicians' Committee for Responsible Medicine, and an Adjunct Associate Professor of Medicine at the George Washington University School of Medicine and Health Sciences.

Dr. Barnard is the author of several books, including *Food for Life*, *Turn Off the Fat Genes*, and *Foods That Fight Pain*. To learn more, visit his website at www.nealbarnard.org.

# Hyla Cass, M.D.

Hyla Cass, M.D. is a nationally recognized expert in the field of integrative medicine and psychiatry, combining the best of leading-edge natural medicine with modern science, in her clinical practice, writings, lectures, and nationwide media appearances. She is currently an Assistant Clinical Professor at UCLA School of Medicine.

Dr. Cass is author of several popular books including *Natural Highs: Supplements, Nutrition and Mind-Body Techniques* and *8 Weeks to Vibrant Health: A Woman's Take-Charge Program to Correct Imbalances, Reclaim Energy, and Restore Well-Being*. For more information on Dr. Cass, and to order her books and supplements, see her website www.drcass.com.

# Lori Shaw-Cohen

Lori Shaw-Cohen is a best-selling author, editor and nationally published journalist, whose work has appeared in numerous publications for almost three decades. Formerly the Managing Editor of 'TEEN Magazine, Ms. Shaw-Cohen's parenting articles and columns, "The Parent Zone" and "Mom Central," have been featured regularly in major newspapers and regional magazines. She has appeared on television and radio, and has spoken at writers' conferences throughout the United States.

In 2005, Ms. Shaw-Cohen co-authored the national bestseller *Home Buying by the Experts*, a book for first-time homeowners. Originally from Southern California (by way of Manhattan), she moved to the Nashville area in 1996 with her husband and three children. Contact her at LoriShawCohen@aol.com.

# Tracy Stevens

Tracy Stevens is an author, editor and book designer. After earning a degree in Writing, Literature and Publishing from Emerson College in 1993, she began work as an editorial assistant in New York. She became the Editorial Director of Quigley Publishing Company in 1997.

Ms. Stevens is a consultant to numerous publishers and authors and has ghostwritten and designed several bestselling books. In addition to her work in the publishing industry, she serves as the executive director of The Hospital to Home Foundation and has worked with other nonprofits worldwide. She has lived in Europe and the Middle East and currently resides in San Diego, California. Contact her at tracy@wordwit.com.

# John Sunyecz, M.D.

Dr. John Sunyecz is a Board Certified OB/GYN in clinical practice in southwest Pennsylvania and the president of MenopauseRx, Inc. He received a Bachelor's of Science cum laude with honors and distinction in Pharmacy from Ohio State University, where he also attended medical school. Upon graduating cum laude from medical school he completed a residency program in Gynecology and Reproductive Sciences at Magee Women's Hospital in Pittsburgh, Pennsylvania, where he also served as Chief Resident.

His gynecological practice and pharmacy background provided the impetus for MenopauseRx, Inc. By providing menopause and perimenopause education and treatment options, MenopauseRx, Inc. has provided information to more than one million women since 1998. Contact Dr. Sunyecz at sunyecz@menopauserx.com

## James Tsai, L.Ac.

Dr. Tsai graduated with honors from Shandong Medical University in China, where he studied western medicine. While practicing as a surgeon at Qian Fe Shan General Hospital, Dr. Tsai experienced the efficacy of acupuncture and Chinese herbs. Consequently, he chose Traditional Chinese Medicine (TCM) for additional study. He completed his TCM training at Jining Medical College.

Dr. Tsai established his private practice in Carlsbad, California in 1988. He combines both western and Chinese medical knowledge to provide the best of both sciences to his patients. Dr. Tsai is a member of the faculty at Pacific College, where he teaches Diagnosis and Evaluation and is a clinical supervisor. Contact Dr. Tsai at (760) 720-7367.

## Andrew Wen, L.Ac.

Andrew Wen was born and raised in Taipei, Taiwan, where he was exposed to Chinese Medicine at an early age. He graduated from The University of California, Irvine, with a Bachelor of Arts Degree in Psychology. In 1999, he obtained certification as a Clinical Hypnotherapist from the United International Hypnosis Institution. He earned his Master's Degree in Traditional Oriental Medicine from Pacific College. He is a practicing National & State Licensed Acupuncturist and Herbalist in California and Arizona. In addition, he practices and has taught the art of Tai Chi as a preventative medicine.

Mr. Wen currently has a private practice in Anthem, Arizona. For more information, please visit www.anthemacupuncture.com

# I*ndex

## A

# B

# C

# D

# E

# M

# N

# O

# P

# Q

# R

# S

## T

## CREDITS